SCIENTIFIC AMERICAN EXPLORES BIG IDEAS

The Future of Medicine

The Editors of *Scientific American*

SCIENTIFIC AMERICAN EDUCATIONAL PUBLISHING
New York

Published in 2024 by Scientific American Educational Publishing
in association with **The Rosen Publishing Group**
2544 Clinton Street, Buffalo, NY 14224

Contains material from Scientific American®, a division of Springer Nature America, Inc., reprinted by permission, as well as original material from The Rosen Publishing Group®.

First Edition

Scientific American
Lisa Pallatroni: Project Editor

Rosen Publishing
Michael Hessel-Mial: Compiling Editor
Michael Moy: Senior Graphic Designer

Cataloging-in-Publication Data
Names: Scientific American, inc., editor.
Title: The future of medicine / the editors of Scientific American.
Description: First edition. | New York : Scientific American Educational Publishing, 2024. | Series: Scientific American explores big ideas | Includes bibliographical references and index. | Audience: Grades 10-12
Identifiers: LCCN 2023036929 | ISBN 9781725350465 (library binding) | ISBN 9781725350458 (paperback) | ISBN 9781725350472 (ebook)
Subjects: LCSH: Medical innovations–Juvenile literature. | Social medicine–Juvenile literature. | Medical informatics–Juvenile literature. | Biomedical engineering–Juvenile literature.
Classification: LCC RA418.5.M4 F88 2024 | DDC 610.285–dc23/eng/20230901
LC record available at https://lccn.loc.gov/2023036929

Manufactured in the United States of America
Websites listed were live at the time of publication.

Cover: PopTika/Shutterstock.com

CPSIA Compliance Information: Batch # CWSA24.
For Further Information contact Rosen Publishing at 1-800-237-9932.

CONTENTS

Introduction 6

Section 1: AI and Medical Technology 7

1.1 An Innovative Robotic Exosuit Boosts both Walking and Running 8
By Jeremy Hsu

1.2 A New Type of Visual Prosthesis 12
By Stephen L. Macknik

1.3 The Surgical Singularity Is Approaching 15
By Sandip S. Panesar

1.4 Neck-Zapping Gadget Reduced All-Nighter Fatigue in New Study 19
By Maddie Bender

1.5 Experimental Brain Implant Could Personalize Depression Therapy 23
By Gary Stix

1.6 AI in Medicine Is Overhyped 26
By Visar Berisha, Julie Liss

Section 2: Medical Treatments Reimagined 30

2.1 Can Hearing Be Restored by Making the Brain More Childlike? 31
By Mo Costandi

2.2 How Virtual Reality Will Transform Medicine 34
By Claudia Wallis

2.3 Can 3-D Printing Produce Lung and Liver Tissue for Transplants? 37
By Starre Vartan

2.4 The Case for Fewer Heart Procedures 41
By Claudia Wallis

2.5 A Breakthrough in Genetic Medicine for Rare Diseases 44
By Lydia Denworth

Section 3: Drug Development and Delivery 55

3.1 A Better Pill—Internal Delivery Devices May Help Patients Take Their Medicine 56
By Knvul Sheikh

3.2 How Nanotech Powers Precision Medicine 60
By Robert Langer

3.3 Tiny, Tumbling Origami Robots Could Help with Targeted Drug Delivery 63
By Fionna M. D. Samuels

3.4 Hope for New Drugs Arises from the Sea 66
By Stephanie Stone

Section 4: Science Evaluates Alternative Medicine 74

4.1 Drug Developers Take a Second Look at Herbal Medicines 75
By Brendan Borrell

4.2 Traditional Medicine from Southern Mexico Offers Help with Addiction 85
By Peter H. Addy, Ana Elda Maqueda

4.3 Anti-Vaxxers Are Here to Stay 90
By Beth S. Linas

4.4 The World Health Organization Gives the Nod to Traditional Chinese Medicine. Bad Idea 94
By The Editors

Section 5: Reproductive and Sexual Health 97

5.1 Maternal Health Care Is Disappearing in Rural America 98
By Dina Fine Maron

5.2 Abortion Bans Based on So-Called "Science" Are Fraudulent 104
By Nicole M. Baran, Gretchen Goldman, Jane Zelikova

5.3 What the Science on Gender-Affirming Care for Transgender Kids Really Shows 111
By Heather Boerner

5.4 What Scientists Are Learning about Women's Health from Other Female Animals 118
By Barbara Natterson-Horowitz

Section 6: Making Healthcare Equitable 127

6.1 Potential Inequities in New Medical Technologies 128
By Eric B. Kmiec, Jonathan Marron

6.2 Inequality before Birth Contributes to Health Inequality in Adults 132
By Janet Currie

6.3 A Tool Doctors Use Every Day Can Perpetuate Medical Racism 145
By Ashley Andreou

6.4 Antifatness in the Surgical Setting 150
By Ashley Andreou

Glossary 155

Further Information 157

Citations 158

Index 159

INTRODUCTION

The healing arts are an area where basic and applied science come together. Fundamental research into the molecule and the cell might take decades, but it eventually arrives at treatments that save lives. Likewise, as new technologies emerge on the scene, people find unexpected ways for them to treat the human body. In the last decade, medicine has gone through such important scientific and social changes.

The most commonly cited example of medical innovation is the rise of medical devices: new ways of testing, treating, interfacing with the body, and sharing medical data. Such devices also come alongside the ongoing revolutions in artificial intelligence and virtual reality. But devices only scratch the surface. Recent novel treatments in drug development, surgery, genetic therapy, and prosthetics may yet solve chronic and/or deadly health issues once deemed impossible to treat. Advances in gene therapy and nanoscale drug delivery are especially exciting examples of long-coming and revolutionary advances.

At the same time, researchers are more widely discussing the social dimensions of human health, including areas researchers have neglected to explore. Reproductive health is one such example: fertility and birth benefit from new studies, while also being subject to a wave of restrictive reproductive health laws that impact people's lives. Similarly, the health impacts of racism and other oppressions are demonstrated with concrete data.

The articles in this title are organized into six sections in the following areas: "AI and Medical Technology," "Medical Treatments Reimagined," "Drug Development and Delivery," "Science Evaluates Alternative Medicine," "Reproductive and Sexual Health," and "Making Healthcare Equitable." Cancer, a very important topic, can be explored in a separate volume. In these articles, readers will find that future medicine will look quite different from before and will include insights on health and wellness that have at times been neglected.

Section 1: AI and Medical Technology

1.1 An Innovative Robotic Exosuit Boosts both Walking and Running
By Jeremy Hsu

1.2 A New Type of Visual Prosthesis
By Stephen L. Macknik

1.3 The Surgical Singularity Is Approaching
By Sandip S. Panesar

1.4 Neck-Zapping Gadget Reduced All-Nighter Fatigue in New Study
By Maddie Bender

1.5 Experimental Brain Implant Could Personalize Depression Therapy
By Gary Stix

1.6 AI in Medicine Is Overhyped
By Visar Berisha, Julie Liss

An Innovative Robotic Exosuit Boosts both Walking and Running

By Jeremy Hsu

A pair of fitted shorts may not look much like the high-tech robotic exoskeletons of Hollywood films. But this seemingly simple device, which tugs on the wearer's legs with each step, probably represents the first exosuit capable of significantly assisting humans in both walking and running.

Until recently, no exosuit design had succeeded in reducing the amount of energy required for both types of motion. Earlier generations of such suits, also known as wearable robots, had stumbled in that challenge because of the different biomechanical actions required for walking versus running. Now researchers have developed a soft device that can automatically detect whether the wearer is walking or running and provide the appropriate assistance for either movement.

"After wearing the system for 15 minutes or so, you start to question if it's really helping at all, because you just feel like you're walking," says David Perry, a robotics engineer at the Wyss Institute for Biologically Inspired Engineering at Harvard University. "Once you shut it off, however, your legs suddenly feel heavy, and you realize how much it was helping. It's a lot like stepping off the end of one of those moving sidewalks at the airport."

To quantify the difference between moving with pure leg power and using robotic assistance, the researchers put wearers on a treadmill and calculated how much oxygen they consumed while breathing, a measure known as metabolic cost. The exosuit showed it could reduce the metabolic costs of walking by 9 percent and of running by 4 percent. Such effects, the researchers say, are equivalent to feeling 16.3 pounds lighter while walking and 12.6 pounds lighter while running. That result could benefit anyone who needs to travel quickly across long distances on foot: rescue workers searching a large disaster area, U.S. Army soldiers or Marines on the march, or even hikers out for fun. It could also provide steady medical assistance to people with illnesses or injuries that restrict walking.

Perry and his colleagues detailed their prototype in a paper published this week in *Science*. The wearable robot relies on soft textile materials and weighs just 11 pounds—a relatively low weight that helps reduce the metabolic cost of running with an extra load. Electric motors worn on the lower back apply force to cables connected to soft leg wraps worn around the thigh of each leg. A battery strapped around the waist provides enough power to help the wearer cover about five miles between charges.

Previous studies have tested portable hip- and ankle-assist devices, finding the latter can help with walking and the former can do so with either walking or running. But the scientists who developed the new exosuit say no individual apparatus until this one has demonstrated the ability to aid both types of motion. "This study builds upon the research team's prior success in developing ankle-assist devices by showing benefits can also be achieved through hip assistance," says Karl Zelik, an assistant professor of mechanical engineering at Vanderbilt University and chief scientific officer at HeroWear, a company that is currently developing lift-assist exosuits. As an expert who did not participate in the recent study, he described its results as "promising."

To help the exosuit automatically switch between walking and running modes, the team installed sensors capable of measuring force and angular motion. It trained a control algorithm to detect walking and running patterns, based on feedback from these sensors. The algorithm eventually learned to tell the difference between how the human body's center of mass moves while walking—in which it acts like an "inverted pendulum," where the hip swings over the planted foot with each forward step—and while running—in which it does so like a "spring-mass" system, where each leg bounces in the manner of a spring attached to the hip.

Beyond the main treadmill experiments, which took place at a minimal incline and constant speed, one male study participant performed additional treadmill testing that mimicked more realistic conditions. The results suggest that the exosuit also helps with uphill walking and with running at varying speeds on a flat surface, says Philippe Malcolm, an assistant professor of biomechanics at the University of Nebraska Omaha and a co-author on the study. "The exciting progress we have made and results we see in this study set up other studies where we can evaluate the device in other outdoor environments, such as hilly and mountainous terrain," Malcolm says.

Much original funding for the exosuit came from the U.S. Defense Advanced Research Projects Agency, through its Warrior Web program, which is aimed at lightening the load for U.S. troops during marches or foot patrols. Because most American soldiers are male, the system's early design and testing centered on the body shapes of men. But the researchers have been developing new versions of the exosuit for women and a broader range of possible wearers, such as those with a variety of disabilities.

Perry and his Harvard colleagues have filed patents on exosuit components and established a licensing agreement with ReWalk Robotics, a medical device company focused on bionic systems. The company has already released one commercial ankle device to help rehabilitate stroke patients and is exploring medical applications based on the hip exosuit system. The researchers are also developing a new version of the exosuit that will weigh 60 percent as much as the current model and will tailor its assistance to best fit each individual wearer's shape and gait.

Personalized gait assistance is particularly difficult in the case of stroke patients or elderly people, who walk and run in less steady and predictable patterns, says José Pons, scientific chair for the Legs + Walking Lab at Shirley Ryan AbilityLab, a translational research hospital in Chicago. He was not involved in the new research but did write an opinion article on the study in the same issue of *Science*. Even the gait-detecting algorithms in advanced exosuits such as this one may find it challenging to detect when less predictable movement is about to shift. "Ideally, the movement intent should be detected before the movement is actually executed so that assistance can be synchronized to the desired movement," Pons says. "Otherwise, the assistance could be felt as opposing the movement rather than assisting it." In his opinion article, Pons suggested that instead of relying on algorithms, future exosuits will need new neural interfaces to directly detect human intentions through nervous-system signals. Technology like that, he says, could help exosuits take their next big step forward.

About the Author

Jeremy Hsu is a New York City–based writer who has contributed to publications such as Scientific American, IEEE Spectrum, Undark Magazine *and* Wired.

A New Type of Visual Prosthesis

By Stephen L. Macknik

In normal vision, light falls on the retinas inside the eyes, and is immediately transduced into electrochemical signals before being uploaded to the brain through the optic nerves. So you do not see light itself, but the brain's interpretation of electrochemical signals in the visual parts of the brain. It follows that, if your eyes do not work, but your brain is stimulated *just so*, your visual neurons will activate (and you will be able to see) just the same as if your eyes were in perfect condition.

Sounds easy, but can we do that? Building on decades of research in visual neuroscience, my lab, in collaboration with Susana Martinez-Conde's, has now conducted some of the studies that validate this idea, completing some of the most important preliminary steps towards a new kind of visual prosthetic.

Francis Collins, the Director of the National Institutes of Health, has just posted a blog that highlights our approach. He took notice of our work when we first presented it at this year's meeting for the Principal Investigators of the BRAIN Initiative–the NIH led government funding initiative meant to spur research along on topics like brain implants. The BRAIN Initiative funds several agencies including the NIH, including the National Science Foundation, who kindly funded the grant driving our research thus far.

Our starting premise is that vision is fundamentally a thumbnail sketch. Even if 99.9% of your retina works fine, but the central 1/1000th of your visual field is broken, you will be legally blind. That central 0.1% of your visual field is about the same size as your thumbnail held up at arm's length. Because that central 0.1% of the retina is the visual sweet spot, it is the place where the visual magic happens. In fact, much of the remaining 99.9% of the retina's main job is to help you detect where to move your eyes next. This means that we need to restore central vision in the blind, or we are not really restoring functional vision at all.

In addition, we also need to achieve prosthetic vision with the same acuity as normal vision, or patients will still be visually impaired. How good is good enough? The answer is in the stars. Go outside on a clear night, look up, and find the stars in the sky. Seems counterintuitive, but the biggest and the smallest-looking stars in the sky are actually the same size from the point of view of your retinal photoreceptors. Because all stars are so far away, the light that reaches Earth from each of them and falls on your retina subtends an area smaller than that of a single photoreceptor. But because of scatter in the atmosphere (and especially in your eye), brighter stars activate more photoreceptors, and therefore seem bigger than dimmer stars. Therefore, the dimmest star in the sky is the smallest thing you can possibly see. If we can prosthetically restore vision of objects of that size, then we can restore vision of *any* objects in the world—which for many patients will be life-changing and worth risking brain surgery.

Our recent research shows that it is possible to stimulate the visual brain at a specific point with enough precision to prosthetically evoke a single star in the sky, at maximal contrast, without stimulating unwanted neurons. That is what it means to stimulate the brain—*just so*—and restore the building blocks of vision.

There are two main steps to our project:

First, to stimulate a stage of visual processing with synaptic precision, just as the natural visual system does it, we need a way to activate neurons in the visual system prosthetically. We do this by injecting a custom virus into the region of the brain where the optic nerves first connect within the center of the brain. The virus injects genes into those cells and changes them into photoreceptors: now they are excitable by light. Because these neurons reach all the way to the visual cortex at the very back of the brain, and because they are laid out in a map that matches the visual world, we can stimulate their synaptic connections precisely with a video projector to recreate how they would react to real incoming visual inputs. We then target the central visual neurons and ultimately restore vision. That is the essence of our planned visual prosthetic.

Second, stimulating neurons without monitoring the effects of the stimulation will not be sufficient. We will also need to read-out the effects of our stimulation in real time, to make power adjustments as a function of the variability inherent to neuronal firing. To restore vision means to account for the regulatory mechanisms that keep the visual system calibrated at all times.

To accomplish this, we will inject more virus, now in the visual cortex, to make those neurons bioluminescent, so that they blink when they are active. By using many differently colored bioluminescent proteins, the neurons will have all sorts of different colors, meaning that we will be able to read-out their activity with a color camera–just like the tiny one on your cell phone.

Third, we will need to build a video projector/color camera that can be implanted in the brain. This is a relatively straightforward engineering task, comparable to or simpler than designing a smart phone. The next several years will reveal whether we can capitalize on these advances, to go from understanding the fundamental building blocks of prosthetic vision to making a functional high-quality visual prosthetic. We will keep you apprised of our progress along the way.

The views expressed are those of the author(s) and are not necessarily those of Scientific American.

About the Author

Stephen L. Macknik is a professor of opthalmology, neurology, and physiology and pharmacology at SUNY Downstate Medical Center in Brooklyn, N.Y. Along with Susana Martinez-Conde and Sandra Blakeslee, he is author of the Prisma Prize-winning Sleights of Mind. *Their book* Champions of Illusion *was published by Scientific American/Farrar, Straus and Giroux in 2017.*

The Surgical Singularity Is Approaching

By Sandip S. Panesar

Those keeping abreast of the latest medical developments may be aware of the buzz surrounding applications of artificial intelligence (AI) to medical tasks. To date, these have mainly involved application of computer algorithms to clinical data such as x-rays, images or text-based medical records, to diagnose disease. The sensationalism has largely arisen due to the fact that in some instances, these algorithms have met or exceeded capabilities of a specialist physician for particular diagnostic tasks.

With these early accomplishments, a question arises as to how the introduction of clinically viable AI may affect the role of human physicians in the future. Being at a primitive stage and lacking widespread real-world application, the topic remains speculative at present. Much of the debate, however, concerns the effect of AI upon non-interventionalists,* whose primary role is to diagnose and treat diseases non-invasively. An interventionalist (i.e., a surgeon) may therefore wonder how the "AI revolution" may affect him or her; after all, an algorithm cannot perform a heart bypass or remove a brain tumor.

In 2016, the Smart Tissue Anastomosis Robot (STAR), an autonomous surgical robot, underwent experimental trials in animals. The robot, which utilized "smart sensing" apparatus including cameras and mechanical sensors, along with AI-control algorithms, outperformed human surgeons at certain tasks, including joining intestine in a living animal *without direct human intervention*.

This was not the first time that AI-controlled robots have experimentally outperformed humans at single surgical tasks such as knot-tying. The closest things to commercially available "autonomous" surgical robots are devices that use external radiation beams to treat cancers (not in direct contact with human tissue) or those offering *reduced* human input for tasks involving rigid, fixed tissues (i.e., bones) for joint replacements.

A mammal's abdomen is soft, deformable, delicate and contains blood vessels and organs at great risk of damage during surgery. STAR had to perform multiple real-time tasks simultaneously, while minimizing risk of collateral damage: "seeing" the environment which it was working in, "sensing" the features of the tissue upon which it was operating and "reacting" to environmental changes as they occurred, effectively mimicking human surgeons' "judgment" in addition to their physical skill.

In their *Science Translational Medicine* paper, the authors noted: "The intent of this demonstration of feasibility in soft tissue surgery was not to replace surgeons but to expand human capacity and capability through enhanced vision, dexterity, and complementary machine intelligence for improved surgical outcomes, safety, and patient access."

Surgical robots have existed for over 30 years and have become widely used by certain specialties because of their technical benefits, which augment human capabilities. These include fatigue resistance, increased range of motion and resistance to shaking. Commercial surgical robot designs utilize a "master-and-slave" arrangement; a human surgeon (master) controls the robot (slave), situated near the patient and a few feet away from the operator, in real time. The technical benefits of using surgical robots have translated into improved outcomes and reduced complications for certain procedures such as prostate surgery.

At present, the costs of purchasing ($1 million to $2.5 million) and maintaining robotic surgical devices are cited as a barrier to their widespread use. Robotic surgical procedures are often more expensive than traditional ones, given the specialized equipment required for the robot. Institutions purchasing these devices must maintain a high volume of cases to recover outlays. Nevertheless, because of the technical advantages of such systems, which include a lower complication rate and better removal of diseased tissue, studies have demonstrated a reduction in overall costs to health care systems for robotic surgery for certain diseases such as prostate cancer.

It is therefore reasonable to predict an evolving symbiosis between the benefits already demonstrated by surgical robots, with the nascent advantages of medical AI. Given further development, we may soon see autonomous surgical robots with capacity to perform complex soft-tissue surgical procedures faster, more accurately and with fewer complications than human surgeons.

If these devices are tested by trial in humans, and the advantages are confirmed, it is also not unreasonable to envision a scenario where continuous technological refinement driven by clinical demand leads to drastic cost reductions for purchasing autonomous surgical devices.

A phenomenon where technological advancement produces real-life cost reductions was described by Gordon Moore, of Fairchild Semiconductor and Intel in the 1960s: With advances in semiconductor technology, Moore predicted that the number of transistors held per square inch of circuit board would double every two years. A medically related example of Moore's Law is provided by the Human Genome Project: In 2001, cost to sequence a single genome was U.S. $100 million.

With improving sequencing technology, costs began to drop in line with Moore's law until 2008. That year, "next generation" sequencing technology was introduced, resulting in cost decreases betraying Moore's law. Sequencing cost per genome plummeted to U.S. $1,000, or 1/100,000 of its initial cost by 2017. In 2018, companies such as 23andme offer personalized genome sequencing kits over the internet for under U.S. $100.

Technological refinement and cost reductions may therefore enable widespread adoption of autonomous surgical robots. A "technological singularity" is a hypothesis that the invention of an artificial superintelligence will result in exponential technological growth, producing unfathomable changes to human civilization. As clinically capable, AI-controlled surgical robots may soon offer technical and economic advantages over human surgeons, a "surgical singularity" may therefore occur when capable, cheap and technically superior autonomous robots are introduced.

It is possible that these devices will transform the technical practice of surgery by enabling optimized removal of diseased tissues, faster operative times and better access to hard-to-reach body areas. These technical benefits will translate into improved survival and fewer complications for patients.

Debate regarding the future role of AI in health care should therefore be extended to include AI-enhanced interventional devices. The issue of how these devices will affect the role of surgeons should be considered and incorporated into any future operating frameworks. An ideal outcome is the augmentation of human surgical capability using AI and robotics, resulting in significantly improved patient care. Aside from encouraging the technical development of these devices, further work should be done regarding the potential impact in terms of workload, regulatory frameworks and the ethical and insurance implications that these devices may have upon surgical practice.

**Physicians can roughly be categorized as non-interventionalists or interventionalists: Non-interventional specialties include diagnostic radiology, pathology, oncology, psychiatry and neurology among many others concerned with the diagnosis and/or pharmaceutical treatment of medical conditions. Interventionalists are surgeons whose task is the physical removal of pathology, or reconstruction of tissues via cutting and suturing, underpinned by their manual dexterity.*

The views expressed are those of the author(s) and are not necessarily those of Scientific American.

About the Author

Sandip S. Panesar is a postdoctoral research fellow in neurosurgery at Stanford University.

Neck-Zapping Gadget Reduced All-Nighter Fatigue in New Study

By Maddie Bender

Instead of reaching for a cup of coffee during a graveyard shift, workers might one day hold an electric-razor-sized device to their necks. After a couple of minutes they would emerge refreshed and awake from this experience, which could come to be known as a "vagus nerve break."

The device, called gammaCore, sends a series of vibrating bursts of low-voltage electricity, each lasting a millisecond, to the side of the neck. It is meant to stimulate part of the vagus nerve, a connector between brain and body, and cause the release of wakefulness chemicals.

Research on a way to keep people awake and alert with electricity began after scientists affiliated and contracted with the Air Force noted that participants who had electrodes placed onto their scalps to deliver a current were able to lower fatigue and improve their performance on attention tasks. This setup is not easy to re-create outside of a lab, but if it were, it could offer an alternative to caffeine or amphetamine stimulants, also known as "go pills," which are still prescribed to U.S. Air Force soldiers.

Looking for a more direct and side-effect-free solution led researchers to the vagus nerve. Surgical implants that stimulate the nerve have been used to prevent seizures in people with epilepsy since 1988, and some of these patients have found that the implant helped them manage their headaches and pain. Other studies have found that implanted vagus nerve stimulation improved memory and cognition in both humans and animals.

New research provides confirmation that handheld vagus nerve stimulation does what scientists thought it might: gammaCore helped members of the Air Force perform better and feel less fatigued when pulling an all-nighter. Results from the study were published today in the journal *Communications Biology*.

Many thought stimulating the vagus nerve without needles or surgery was impossible before the technology was invented a decade ago, says Peter Staats, chief medical officer and co-founder of electroCore, the company that makes gammaCore. The handheld device works by touching conductive gel on the skin's surface, and it was first approved to treat cluster headaches in adults in 2017. Since then, its use has been expanded to include adult and adolescent migraines, and it has received emergency use authorization for asthma worsened by COVID-19 in adults. The device is covered by several major pharmacy benefit managers when it is prescribed, and its list price is $1,750, though the company says it has been offering gammaCore to all customers for $1,250 for now. (An electroCore spokesperson notes the newest model can cost as low as $399 for three months of treatment.)

Vagus nerve stimulation is a popular target for bioelectronic medicine because of the direct links between the nerve and many of the body's organs. Stephen Silberstein, a neurology professor at Thomas Jefferson University and director of the Jefferson Headache Center, compares the vagus nerve to a major transportation hub such as Grand Central Terminal in New York City, where hopping on a train or subway can send a commuter anywhere in the metropolitan area. Similarly, different types of fibers travel to different places, including a part of the brain called the locus coeruleus. There, the brain produces norepinephrine, a fight-or-flight chemical that increases alertness and decreases pain and tiredness.

In the study, researchers observed 40 active-duty soldiers from an Air Force base as they stayed awake for 34 hours, during which time they completed cognitive tests and reported their mood and level of fatigue. Half of the participants used gammaCore for eight minutes near the beginning of testing, while the other half were given a sham device that looked and felt like the real deal but did not provide an electrical current. Those in the group that received the real vagus nerve stimulation stuck more closely to their baseline performance as the night wore on and reported less fatigue over time than the other group.

"It's exciting to us that not only do they perform better, but they also perceive that they're performing better and that they feel less tired," says Richard McKinley, a co-author of the study and a biomedical engineer at the Air Force Research Laboratory. He says that improvements in mood and energy level could motivate the soldiers to use a device like this outside of a paid study.

While the two groups performed similarly over time on some portions of the cognitive testing, hours later, the participants who used gammaCore showed less performance decline in perception-related tasks–taking in and synthesizing audio, visual or other kinds of information.

Past research on gammaCore and vagus nerve stimulation has targeted populations with chronic and often debilitating conditions such as rheumatoid arthritis, migraine headaches and epilepsy. This new work is leading the charge to use this therapy on healthy people for performance enhancement, Staats and the study's authors say.

"Much of what we do in Western medicine is: we try to help people who have already got diseases," Staats says. "We spend less effort thinking about health regimens or 'How do we avoid development of diseases?' or 'How do we optimize ourselves?'"

Silberstein, who was not involved in the study, says this device could help a wide range of sleep-deprived individuals, from Air Force pilots to doctors to college students writing last-minute papers.

Another group that might benefit from the research is astronauts. Lindsey McIntire, the paper's first author and a scientist at the defense-contracted company Infoscitex, says that NASA provided some of the study's funding because astronauts often sleep in extreme and unfamiliar environments, leading to less restful slumber. Finding a long-lasting solution to fatigue would keep people happier, healthier and more focused on their tasks in space.

Eric Chang, an assistant professor at the Feinstein Institutes for Medical Research, who was also not involved in the research, says its findings may not be generalizable to people who are not continuously sleep-deprived for 34 straight hours, as the participants were. He adds that the study reports a "specific, small result" that is in line with other vagus-nerve-stimulation studies.

McIntire notes that differences in performance between the gammaCore and placebo groups that may appear small—such as in the multitasking test—can have big implications. "Performance for the active group declined 5 percent, but it declined to 15 percent for [the placebo group]," she says. "That's mistakes, and in certain fields like medicine and the military and transportation, that can equal lives." The authors are also planning research to examine effects in people with milder sleep deprivation.

McIntire says future studies need to be done before gammaCore can be recommended to soldiers and workers for off-label use, including testing it against caffeine and other conventional stimulants. McKinley adds that concurrent studies in animals are double-checking the effect's mechanism, and he is also preparing to submit research on vagus nerve stimulation to boost learning rates and retention.

GammaCore owes its invention to the relatively new field of bioelectric medicine, a discipline that uses electricity to hack into the body's signaling system to treat disease. Bioelectronic medicine has shown promise in treating autoimmune diseases such as lupus through vagus nerve stimulation. Tiredness, pain, inflammation—future "vagus nerve breaks" could target them all.

About the Author

Maddie Bender is a science writer and podcaster based in Boston, Mass. Follow her on Twitter @MaddieOBender.

Experimental Brain Implant Could Personalize Depression Therapy

By Gary Stix

Sarah remembers what it was like both before and after the treatment. The 36-year old vividly recalls how, after her depression lifted, she had to readapt to performing the tasks other people do routinely each day. Even the simple act of looking at a menu took readjustment.

"I also had to learn, relearn," she said at a press briefing, "how to actually have opinions about things and actually pick something on a menu and order it and not just go along with what everyone else wanted. Because I was so used to the fact that I couldn't make decisions, that [ability], over the last five years...., just atrophied and disappeared."

Sarah's intractable depression, which had not responded even to electroconvulsive therapy, yielded after an experimental treatment conducted at the University of California, San Francisco. The treatment detects depression-related brain activity and then applies electrical stimulation at a targeted location to relieve symptoms. The device used for the procedure has already been approved for treating epilepsy by providing brain stimulation after it registers electrical patterns that predict an oncoming seizure.

In the October 4 study in *Nature Medicine*, the researchers describe how they set about to find a stimulation site using electrodes to probe emotion circuitry in Sarah's brain. As they looked, they found that one site might lower anxiety and that another might increase energy levels.

When the team activated a site deep in Sarah's brain in a reward-related area called the ventral striatum, she had an immediate reaction. Sarah was doing needlework during one session to distract herself from negative thoughts when a stimulus was applied to that spot. Her mood changed quickly. In a U.C.S.F. article about the treatment, she recounted her surprise at feeling that she was enjoying what she was doing–experiencing, in fact, a sense of "glee and happiness."

The researchers also wanted to know when to provide a stimulus. Previous research on activating neural circuits to relieve depression using other deep-brain stimulation (DBS) techniques have met with mixed results. Earlier attempts did not map the brain to take into account the fact that depression may vary among individuals.

These efforts also applied continuous stimulation. The U.C.S.F. researchers suspect that the effectiveness of this type of treatment depends on knowing when an electrode should be activated in anticipation of symptoms growing more severe, similar to the approach taken with epilepsy.

They looked for what they call a "biomarker" that could supply such an alert. They found it in the amygdala, which mediates emotional processes and is also connected to the striatum. High-frequency neural activity–"gamma oscillations"–in the amygdala indicated when symptoms were about to get worse.

Last year the team implanted the about $30,000 epilepsy device, Neuropace RNS, in the right hemisphere of Sarah's brain. An electrical wire goes to the amygdala to detect gamma activity. When present, a warning flashes back to a thin metal disk placed in the skull. The disk, a neurostimulator, then transmits a signal along a separate wire to the striatum to tamp down feelings of sadness and depression.

Stimulation is applied in a short six-second burst and then turns off until another gamma warning is received. This intermittent switching on adds up to no more than 30 minutes a day. But for Sarah, it has made a difference. "The device has kept my depression at bay," Sarah said at the press briefing, "allowing me to return to my best self and rebuild a life worth living."

When tried with new patients, the therapy will again be personalized. Others will also undergo the process of electrical probing to look for brain stimulation areas most suited to their depression. But the challenges accompanying Sarah's case make the U.C.S.F. researchers optimistic. "We didn't know if we were going to be able to treat her depression at all because it was so severe," said Katherine Scangos, a U.C.S.F. physician and lead author of the *Nature Medicine* paper, at the press briefing.

Longtime DBS researchers also took notice. "This is an interesting and important proof of principle case," says Helen Mayberg, a neurologist at the Icahn School of medicine at Mount Sinai, who has been a pioneer in earlier DBS studies for depression and was not involved in the new study. "Time will tell if this approach substantively improves on simpler open-loop strategies [without biomarkers]."

Andres Lozano, a professor of neurosurgery at the University of Toronto and a collaborator of Mayberg's, who was also not involved in the *Nature Medicine* paper, says that the work is an "exciting finding that leads to a more personalized and 'just in time' approach to delivering brain stimulation in depression when and where it is needed." He adds that "several questions remain, including the generalizability of these biomarkers across patients and whether the application of stimulation produces more than merely acute changes but indeed an enduring benefit."

Sarah is just one patient. The study she enrolled in was a "proof of concept"–what researchers call an "*n* of one." "We're still learning; we're at the very, very beginning of trying to understand how this works," says U.C.S.F. neurosurgeon Edward Chang, who is co-senior author of the study. U.C.S.F. is in the process of lining up 11 additional patients. The new research could ultimately provide a better idea of whether targeting just the right brain circuit can lift the penumbra that hangs over a severely depressed person.

About the Author

Gary Stix is a senior editor at Scientific American.

AI in Medicine Is Overhyped

By Visar Berisha, Julie Liss

We use tools that rely on artificial intelligence (AI) every day, with voice assistants like Alexa and Siri being among the most common. These consumer products work reasonably well—Siri understands most of what we say—but they are by no means perfect. We accept their limitations and adapt how we use them until they get the right answer, or we give up. After all, the consequences of Siri or Alexa misunderstanding a user request are usually minor.

However, mistakes by AI models that support doctors' clinical decisions can mean life or death. Therefore, it's critical that we understand how well these models work before deploying them. Published reports of this technology currently paint a too-optimistic picture of its accuracy, which at times translates to sensationalized stories in the press. Media are rife with discussions of algorithms that can diagnose early Alzheimer's disease with up to 74 percent accuracy or that are more accurate than clinicians. The scientific papers detailing such advances may become foundations for new companies, new investments and lines of research, and large-scale implementations in hospital systems. In most cases, the technology is not ready for deployment.

Here's why: As researchers feed data into AI models, the models are expected to become more accurate, or at least not get worse. However, our work and the work of others has identified the opposite, where the reported accuracy in published models decreases with increasing data set size.

The cause of this counterintuitive scenario lies in how the reported accuracy of a model is estimated and reported by scientists. Under best practices, researchers train their AI model on a portion of their data set, holding the rest in a "lockbox." They then use that "held-out" data to test their model for accuracy. For example, say an AI program is being developed to distinguish people with dementia from people without it by analyzing how they speak. The model is developed using training data that consist of spoken language samples and dementia diagnosis labels, to predict whether a person has dementia from their speech. It is then tested against held-out data of the same type to estimate how accurately it will perform. That estimate of accuracy then gets reported in academic publications; the higher the accuracy on the held-out data, the better the scientists say the algorithm performs.

And why does the research say that reported accuracy decreases with increasing data set size? Ideally, the held-out data are never seen by the scientists until the model is completed and fixed. However, scientists may peek at the data, sometimes unintentionally, and modify the model until it yields a high accuracy, a phenomenon known as data leakage. By using the held-out data to modify their model and then to test it, the researchers are virtually guaranteeing the system will correctly predict the held-out data, leading to inflated estimates of the model's true accuracy. Instead, they need to use new data sets for testing, to see if the model is actually learning and can look at something fairly unfamiliar to come up with the right diagnosis.

While these overoptimistic estimates of accuracy get published in the scientific literature, the lower-performing models are stuffed in the proverbial "file drawer," never to be seen by other researchers; or, if they are submitted for publication, they are less likely to be accepted. The impacts of data leakage and publication bias are exceptionally large for models trained and evaluated on small data sets. That is, models trained with small data sets are more likely to report inflated estimates of accuracy; therefore we see this peculiar trend in the published literature where models trained on small data sets report higher accuracy than models trained on large data sets.

We can prevent these issues by being more rigorous about how we validate models and how results are reported in the literature. After determining that development of an AI model is ethical for a particular application, the first question an algorithm designer should ask is "Do we have enough data to model a complex construct like human health?" If the answer is yes, then scientists should spend more time on reliable evaluation of models and less time trying to squeeze every ounce of "accuracy" out of a model. Reliable validation of models begins with ensuring we have representative data. The most challenging problem in AI model development is the design of the training and test data itself. While consumer AI companies opportunistically harvest data, clinical AI models require more care because of the high stakes. Algorithm designers should routinely question the size and composition of the data used to train a model to make sure they are representative of the range of a condition's presentation and of users' demographics. All datasets are imperfect in some ways. Researchers should aim to understand the limitations of the data used to train and evaluate models and the implications of these limitations on model performance.

Unfortunately, there is no silver bullet for reliably validating clinical AI models. Every tool and every clinical population are different. To get to satisfactory validation plans that take into account real-world conditions, clinicians and patients need to be involved early in the design process, with input from stakeholders like the Food and Drug Administration. A broader conversation is more likely to ensure that the training data sets are representative; that the parameters for knowing the model works are relevant; and what the AI tells a clinician is appropriate. There are lessons to be learned from the reproducibility crisis in clinical research, where strategies like pre-registration and patient centeredness in research were proposed as a means of increasing transparency and fostering trust. Similarly, a sociotechnical approach to AI model design recognizes that building trustworthy and responsible AI models for clinical applications is not strictly a technical problem. It requires deep knowledge of the underlying clinical application area, a recognition that these models exist in the context of larger systems, and an understanding of the potential harms if the model performance degrades when deployed.

Without this holistic approach, AI hype will continue. And this is unfortunate because technology has real potential to improve clinical outcomes and extend clinical reach into underserved communities. Adopting a more holistic approach to developing and testing clinical AI models will lead to more nuanced discussions about how well these models can work and their limitations. We think this will ultimately result in the technology reaching its full potential and people benefitting from it.

The authors thank Gautam Dasarathy, Pouria Saidi and Shira Hahn for enlightening conversations on this topic. They helped elucidate some of the points discussed in the article.

This is an opinion and analysis article, and the views expressed by the author or authors are not necessarily those of Scientific American.

About the Authors

Visar Berisha is an associate professor in the College of Engineering and the College of Health Solutions at Arizona State University and a co-founder of Aural Analytics. He is an expert in practical and theoretical machine learning and signal processing with applications to health care.

Julie Liss is a professor and associate dean in the College of Health Solutions at Arizona State University and co-founder of Aural Analytics. She is an expert on speech analytics in the context of neurological health and disease.

Section 2: Medical Treatments Reimagined

2.1 Can Hearing Be Restored by Making the Brain More Childlike?
By Mo Costandi

2.2 How Virtual Reality Will Transform Medicine
By Claudia Wallis

2.3 Can 3-D Printing Produce Lung and Liver Tissue for Transplants?
By Starre Vartan

2.4 The Case for Fewer Heart Procedures
By Claudia Wallis

2.5 A Breakthrough in Genetic Medicine for Rare Diseases
By Lydia Denworth

Can Hearing Be Restored by Making the Brain More Childlike?

By Mo Costandi

You can't teach an old dog new tricks—or can you? Textbooks tell us that early infancy offers a narrow window of opportunity during which sensory experience shapes the way neuronal circuits wire up to process sound and other inputs. A lack of proper stimulation during this "critical period" has a permanent and detrimental effect on brain development.

But new research shows the auditory system in the adult mouse brain can be induced to revert to an immature state similar to that in early infancy, improving the animals' ability to learn new sounds. The findings, published Thursday in *Science*, suggest potential new ways of restoring brain function in human patients with neurological diseases—and of improving adults' ability to learn languages and musical instruments.

In mice, a critical period occurs during which neurons in a portion of the brain's wrinkled outer surface, the cortex, are highly sensitized to processing sound. This state of plasticity allows them to strengthen certain connections within brain circuits, fine-tuning their auditory responses and enhancing their ability to discriminate between different tones. In humans, a comparable critical period may mark the beginning of language acquisition. But heightened plasticity declines rapidly, and this continues throughout life, making it increasingly difficult to learn.

In 2011 Jay Blundon, a developmental neurobiologist at Saint Jude Children's Research Hospital, and his colleagues reported that the critical periods for circuits connecting the auditory cortex and the thalamus occur at about the same time. (The thalamus relays information from the sense organs to the appropriate cortical area). These developmental windows seem to be controlled by a molecule called adenosine, levels of which rise after the critical period closes. This inhibits communication between cells in the two regions.

In the latest study the researchers wanted to determine if halting adenosine signaling would reinstate plasticity in the auditory cortex. In one set of experiments they used microelectrodes to measure how neurons in the auditory cortex of healthy adult mice responded to pure tones. Responses were compared with those from animals genetically engineered to lack the cell surface receptor to which adenosine binds. The analysis revealed cells in the auditory cortex of mice lacking the adenosine receptor responded to a larger range of frequencies than those of the wild-type mice.

To investigate further, Blundon and his colleagues inhibited adenosine signaling in several other ways. They engineered their own strain of mice, whose adenosine receptors could be deleted from thalamus cells when the mice reached maturity. The thalamus sends fibers to the area of the cortex where sounds are processed. This genetic engineering expanded the frequency of sounds to which cells in the auditory cortex were responsive, improving the mice's perception of the sounds and improving their ability to discriminate between similar tones. Blocking adenosine signaling with a drug had the same effect on healthy mice. "This [signaling] mechanism, if blocked, is sufficient to extend critical plasticity to late adulthood," says developmental neurobiologist Stanislav Zakharenko, senior author of the study, adding that the findings could help to make language learning in adults more efficient. "Learning a language is very easy for two- to three-year-olds, but language learning courses for adults aren't very effective, even though adults are still capable of learning other skills effectively," he says. "But if I take a take a language course while inhibiting adenosine production or signaling in the thalamus, I would acquire the information quicker, retain it for longer and maybe lose my accent."

The researchers also believe their findings could offer a new treatment for conditions such as stroke as well as tinnitus, or ringing in the ears. They think drug that blocks adenosine signaling could circumvent stroke damage to the auditory cortex by restoring plasticity, and by "retraining" healthy surrounding areas to respond to sounds normally processed by the damaged areas.

Not everyone is convinced by the results, however. "The range of techniques deployed in this work is very impressive," says neuroscientist Jennifer Linden of the Ear Institute at University College London who was not part of the study. "[But] I am skeptical about the conclusion that disrupting adenosine signaling in the thalamus rejuvenates plasticity in the auditory cortex and improves auditory perception." She says interfering with adenosine signaling could alter the excitability of neurons in the thalamus. That would make it unclear whether the observed changes in plasticity and hearing arise specifically from inhibited adenosine signaling, rather than because of altered activity of another internal cell pathway in the thalamus.

Investigating this question is important because altering the excitability of thalamus neurons might impair auditory perception, Linden adds. "Decades of research have linked increased excitability in auditory brain structures with phantom sound perception in tinnitus," she says. "If disrupting adenosine signaling produces improvements in cortical plasticity but also hearing problems such as tinnitus, then it would not be an effective means of improving auditory perception in humans."

But Blundon and his colleagues stand by their assertions. Increased adenosine, he says, reduces the release of the signaling molecule glutamate in the thalamus, which in turn diminishes the activity of neurons in the auditory cortex. "That decrease in adenosine signaling is sufficient to restore cortical plasticity in adults, while activation of adenosine receptors in juveniles is sufficient to block it," Blundon explains. "We do not claim that other processes that could conceivably alter thalamic excitability have no role in the presence or absence of adult auditory cortex plasticity or changes in auditory perception–though we know of no such processes that have been described, and have ruled some out in our previous publications."

How Virtual Reality Will Transform Medicine

By Claudia Wallis

If you still think of virtual reality as the province of dystopian science fiction and geeky gamers, you had better think again. Faster than you can say "*Ready Player One*," VR is starting to transform our world, and medicine may well be the first sector where the impact is profound. Behavioral neuroscientist Walter Greenleaf of Stanford University has been watching this field develop since the days when VR headsets cost $75,000 and were so heavy, he remembers counterbalancing them with a brick. Today some weigh about a pound and cost less than $200. Gaming and entertainment are driving current sales, but Greenleaf predicts that "the deepest and most significant market will be in clinical care and in improving health and wellness."

Even in the early days, when the user entered a laughably low-resolution world, VR showed great promise. By the mid-1990s research had shown it could distract patients from painful medical procedures and ease anxiety disorders. One initial success was SnowWorld, which immersed burn patients in a cool, frozen landscape where they could lob snowballs at cartoon penguins and snowmen, temporarily blocking out the real world where nurses were scrubbing wounds, stretching scar tissue and gingerly changing dressings. A 2011 study with 54 children in burn units found an up to 44 percent reduction in pain during VR sessions–with the bonus that these injured kids said they had "fun."

Another success came in the wake of 9/11. Psychologist JoAnn Difede of NewYork-Presbyterian/Weill Cornell Medical Center began using VR with World Trade Center survivors suffering from post-traumatic stress disorder (PTSD) and later with soldiers returning from Afghanistan and Iraq.

In Difede's laboratory, I saw the original 9/11 VR program with its scenes of lower Manhattan and the newer Bravemind system, which depicts Iraqi and Afghan locales. Developed with Department of Defense funding by Albert "Skip" Rizzo and Arno Hartholt, both at the University of Southern California, Bravemind is used to treat PTSD at about 100 U.S. sites. The approach is based on exposure therapy, in which patients mentally revisit the source of their trauma guided by a therapist who helps them form a more coherent, less intrusive memory. In VR, patients do not merely reimagine the scene, they are immersed in it.

Difede showed me how therapists can customize scenes in Bravemind to match a patient's experience. A keystroke can change the weather, add the sound of gunfire or the call to prayers. It can detonate a car bomb or ominously empty a marketplace. An optional menu of odors enables the patient to sniff gunpowder or spices through a metal tube. "What you do with exposure therapy is systematically go over the trauma," Difede explains. "We're teaching the brain to process and organize the memory so that it can be filed away and no longer intrudes constantly in the patient's life." The results, after nine to 12 gradually intensifying sessions, can be dramatic. One 2010 study with 20 patients found that 16 no longer met the criteria for PTSD after VR treatment.

Until recently, large-scale studies of VR have been missing in action. This is changing fast with the advent of cheaper, portable systems. Difede, Rizzo and three others just completed a randomized controlled trial with nearly 200 PTSD patients. Expected to be published this year, it may shed light on which patients do best with this high-tech therapy and which do not. In a study with her colleague, burn surgeon Abraham Houng, Difede is aiming to quantify the pain-distraction effects of a successor to SnowWorld called Bear Blast, a charming VR game in which patients toss balls at giggly cartoon bears. They will measure whether burn patients need lower doses of intravenous painkillers while playing.

Greenleaf counts at least 20 clinical arenas, ranging from surgical training to stroke rehabilitation to substance abuse where VR is being applied. It can, for example, help recovering addicts avoid relapses by practicing "refusal skills"–turning down drinks at a virtual bar or heroin at a virtual party. Brain imaging suggests that such scenes can evoke very real cravings, just as Bravemind can evoke the heart-racing panic of a PTSD episode. Researchers foresee a day when VR will help make mental health care cheaper and more accessible, including in rural areas.

In a compelling 2017 paper that reviews 25 years of work, Rizzo and co-author Sebastian Koenig ask whether clinical VR is finally "ready for primetime." If today's larger studies bear out previous findings, the answer seems to be an obvious "yes."

About the Author

Claudia Wallis is an award-winning science journalist whose work has appeared in the New York Times, Time, Fortune *and the* New Republic. *She was science editor at* Time *and managing editor of* Scientific American Mind.

Can 3-D Printing Produce Lung and Liver Tissue for Transplants?

By Starre Vartan

Every day an average of 18 people die waiting for an organ transplant in the United States. Donated organs are tough to come by, which is why many scientists have spent the last two decades trying to create new livers, kidneys, hearts or lungs from scratch. One potential way to craft such delicate structures is 3-D printing with biologically compatible materials, or bioprinting—which has now reportedly produced functional models of lung and liver tissues, with a little help from an unconventional ingredient: food dye.

Would-be organ printers previously have been stymied by the complexity of certain organs. Our lungs and livers, for example, contain physically and biochemically entangled networks of blood vessels and airways (in the lung) or bile ducts (in the liver). Being able to recreate this vasculature—and make the fluid dynamics work so blood and other fluids flow properly—has been an ongoing challenge.

Now, a team of researchers from the University of Washington and Rice University say they have produced functional tissue models using a 3-D printing technique called projection stereolithography. This method exposes thin layers of liquid resin to blue light, which solidifies them into intricate arrangements of hydrogels—gels made up of tangled strings of polymer molecules. These form a structural "scaffolding," into which researchers can implant live cells that enable it do the work of a lung or liver. In the new study the implanted cells survived, and the resulting models of organ tissue demonstrated some functions of the real thing. The results were published last week in *Science*.

"This is definitely a major advance in our ability to create 3-D-printed structures that approximate normal tissue," says Anthony Atala, the director of the Wake Forest Institute for Regenerative Medicine, who was not involved in the new study.

The basic technology of projection stereolithography has been around since the 1980s, but "it wasn't designed with biology in mind; it was used to make plastic structures," says Jordan Miller, assistant professor of bioengineering at Rice's Brown School of Engineering and a co-author of the new paper. The technique can produce finer layers than standard 3-D printing, and is faster, too. "Instead of creating one layer in minutes by extrusion, we can do it in seconds" with stereolithography," Miller says. That speed is crucial: since the printed structure ultimately channels oxygen and nutrients to the cells, faster work means fewer cells die in the process of making it.

But there was a challenge. This type of printing process relies on photoreactor chemicals (ones that respond to light), so that certain preprogrammed areas of the liquid will solidify while other areas remain soft and can later be washed away. Unfortunately, many of these chemicals are carcinogenic. For a 3-D printer to create the fine vasculature an organ requires for nutrient delivery and waste removal, it needs the precision offered by stereolithography; but for transplants it would need safe, water-soluble photoreactors.

So, the researchers had to find a replacement for the proven but toxic chemicals. When Miller and his team guessed food dye might do the trick–they knew it would absorb the right light wavelengths to make the 3-D printing process work, and is relatively biocompatible–they were too impatient to wait for a supplier to ship the ingredient. So, Miller says, "I went to the supermarket, and I bought a kit of food coloring dye that people use to make confectionery."

It worked. First, the team colored liquid polymers with the food dye yellow no. 5, or tartrazine, and then had the printer's projector shine blue light on it. This induced a local chemical reaction that solidified the liquid. Because the printer projected light in a preprogrammed pattern, it created a design that hardened into a thin but tough biological structure. "We were screaming with joy, because it was stunning how simple an idea it was; it immediately enabled us to make this dramatically more complex architecture," Miller says.

Yellow no. 5, found in many snack foods, had another advantage: It easily rinsed off the bioprinted structures, leaving a clear framework ready to nurture whatever cells the scientists filled it with. The traces of the dye that remained were not expected to affect cell health. (Studies suggest yellow no. 5 does not affect sperm count, as has been rumored; it might, however, exacerbate preexisting hyperactive disorders in children.)

To the Test

Although researchers have bioprinted tissues before, they have been unable to keep cells alive long enough. The latest study had to test the newly printed scaffolding in this regard, and red blood cells were a simple way to start.

The team created a scale model of an air sac mimicking a crucial part of a lung's complex vascular network. It included one passage for air and separate channels for blood cells. In a healthy human lung, these two structures exchange oxygen without ever touching. The model performed the same feat, keeping the blood cells alive. It also proved sturdy enough to retain its structure as a simulated "breath" expanded and contracted the printed tissues.

Next, the researchers tested a model of liver tissue. Part of the printing process here included injecting specialized liver cells called hepatocytes into the printed structure. The team implanted the artificial liver tissues into live mice with chronic liver injury, as well as non-injured mice, then tested them. A fully functioning liver has over 500 functions and in this case they examined just one, but it did prove successful–and the hepatocytes survived in the living mice.

The new printing method also produced working intravascular valves, which play a key role in the heart and leg veins. In tests the printed versions maintained their structure as fluid flowed through them, and they kept it from moving backward through the valves.

Printed Organs Open Up

So how long until bioprinted organs are available to those on transplant lists? Scientists still have a lot to figure out–starting with the basics, such as determining the optimal base hydrogel. What kind of protein works best? And should additives such as growth factors be used to speed the process? "Now we can start methodically varying these factors to see which are more important–and asking how this affects the functions of the cells," says paper co-author Kelly Stevens, an assistant professor in the University of Washington's bioengineering and pathology departments. Then there is the question of how best to build the scaffolding, and how much printed material could realistically replace tissue. "Those are questions that this new leap in tech enables us to ask for the first time," Stevens says.

The researchers did not want to be the only ones trying out these possibilities–so they made their technology open-source, allowing other bioengineers to test their own applications. "Bioprinting being open-source really helps to accelerate this technology–it really advances the field faster," Atala says. He plans on applying the findings to a number of organ tissue structures his team is working on.

Other would-be organ-builders can buy specialized printers and inks–Miller and some of the paper's other collaborators have founded a start-up, called Volumetric, to sell these materials–or can replicate the work themselves. Miller says sharing the DIY option was important to him. "We really are excited," he says, "about opening up a new set of design freedoms in bioprinting."

About the Author

Starre Vartan is a science writer and investigative reporter at work on a book challenging cultural myths and health misinformation about women's bodies (Hachette, 2024). She began her career as an environmental geologist in New England, wrote screenplays on science subjects for HBO and CBS, ran a successful blog in the mid-aughts, and has been published in National Geographic, New Scientist, Undark, *CNN and more. A graduate of Syracuse University and Columbia University, she is a dual citizen of the U.S. and Australia and splits her time between the Seattle and Sydney areas.*

The Case for Fewer Heart Procedures

By Claudia Wallis

Modern heart surgery is miraculous. To think a failing aortic valve can be replaced via catheter without even cutting open the chest is to appreciate one of the wonders of 21st-century medicine. But as two recent landmark studies suggest, we may be a bit too avid for cardiac procedures. When it comes to treating some common heart conditions, medication can often get the job done. That was the lesson of the much anticipated ISCHEMIA trial, the results of which were revealed at last November's meeting of the American Heart Association. The study involved 5,179 people with moderate to severe ischemia–insufficient blood flow to the heart–caused by narrowing of the coronary arteries. All participants in ISCHEMIA (International Study of Comparative Health Effectiveness with Medical and Invasive Approaches) got medication optimized for their needs: statins and sometimes additional cholesterol-reducing drugs; aspirin or other blood thinners; plus drugs to lower their blood pressure and heart rate where helpful. Subjects were educated on diet, exercise and relaxation techniques. But half the participants were randomly selected to also be treated with either stents–devices that prop open narrowed vessels–or, if stenting was not possible, with bypass surgery.

Although both procedures are routinely used to treat blocked vessels, researchers found that over a three-year period they offered no advantage over drug therapy alone in reducing the rate of heart attacks, hospitalization for heart failure or chest pain, or cardiac death. Past studies had come to similar conclusions, but this trial was larger and better designed, involving patients with more severe cardiovascular disease–the very patients thought to benefit from an invasive approach. Still, it makes sense that medication works so well: "When you have coronary narrowing, it's not just where you see it; it's all throughout the arteries," explains study chair Judith Hochman, senior associate dean of clinical sciences at NYU

Langone Health. "Medical therapy addresses all of them where stenting addresses only the focal ones."

Where the procedures did outshine drugs was in reducing chest pain, or angina. One out of five patients who had daily or weekly chest pain became angina-free within one year with drug therapy, but that rose to one out of two with the invasive strategy. That finding suggests that people prone to angina might want to opt for a procedure. It's important to note that stents and bypass remain vital therapies for people suffering from heart attacks or unstable angina and those with narrowing of the left main coronary artery—all higher-risk groups not included in this trial.

Another study comparing heart medication with a more invasive treatment yielded similar results. Published last March, the CABANA trial looked at two approaches to atrial fibrillation—bouts of rapid, irregular heartbeats that afflict about 2 percent of adults younger than 65 and 9 percent of seniors in the U.S. The 2,204 patients in the study were randomly assigned to be treated with just medication or with catheter ablation, a procedure in which heat or cold was used to isolate or destroy heart tissue causing the abnormal rhythm. In this study, too, there was no difference between the two groups in mortality or in rates of disabling stroke, serious bleeding or cardiac arrest. Again, there was a difference in terms of symptoms: ablation patients were less likely to have recurrent attacks of A-fib and reported a better quality of life. By some measures ablation also outperformed drugs for patients younger than 65, minorities, and people with heart failure, says cardiologist Douglas Packer of the Mayo Clinic, who led the trial.

The studies should help put more decision-making power into the hands of patients. Rather than being rushed to the "cath lab" for a procedure on pain of death, people can take time to weigh their options. "I think the two studies are, in some senses, are twins," says Stephen Wiviott, a cardiovascular medicine specialist at Brigham and Women's Hospital, who was not involved in either trial. "They are fairly patient-empowering."

The studies' impact will be fascinating to see. At least 500,000 cardiac stent procedures are done annually in the U.S., many on an emergency basis. If doctors simply stopped doing them electively in the least symptomatic patients—those without angina—the U.S. could eliminate about 22,800 procedures a year, saving about $570 million, Hochman says. Ablations may also decline for people with few A-fib symptoms, but Packer says the quality-of-life argument for many patients is strong: "CABANA can't support the notion that people will live longer because of an ablation. It supports the notion that they will live better."

About the Author

Claudia Wallis is an award-winning science journalist whose work has appeared in the New York Times, Time, Fortune *and the* New Republic. *She was science editor at* Time *and managing editor of* Scientific American Mind.

A Breakthrough in Genetic Medicine for Rare Diseases

By Lydia Denworth

At her first birthday, Emma Larson was not walking or standing, but neither are plenty of other kids at that age. She loved the bouncer her parents set up in their Long Island, N.Y., home, and she crawled with gusto. Then, at 13 months, Emma's legs stopped working. Her mother, Dianne Larson, snaps her fingers and says, "It was like that." Emma stopped bouncing. Her legs buckled when she pulled herself up to stand. The change in her crawling was subtler, but when her parents looked at an old video, the difference was obvious–Emma now covered less ground and struggled to hold her head up.

After a barrage of testing, in July 2014 the Larsons learned that Emma had spinal muscular atrophy (SMA), a potentially deadly neurodegenerative disease that strikes mostly children, robbing them of the ability to walk, talk and, in the worst cases, breathe. Her motor neurons were dying because of a severe lack of a protein called SMN (survival motor neuron) in her body. "You go through the darkest of dark periods," Dianne says. But the family was determined to "go down swinging," says Matt Larson, Emma's father. "We were willing to do pretty much anything to combat this terrible disease."

Not far from the Larsons' home, at Cold Spring Harbor Laboratory, biochemist and molecular geneticist Adrian Krainer was engaged in the same fight. He had been investigating the genetic underpinnings of SMA since 2000 and knew the problem was a missing or mutated essential gene, *SMN1*. But he also understood that people carry an inactive and potentially salvageable analogue of that gene, *SMN2*. By 2004 he had joined forces with Frank Bennett of Ionis Pharmaceuticals to try to create a drug capable of altering *SMN2* in SMA patients so that it could ultimately generate functional SMN protein, with the aim of ameliorating the progression of the disease. To that end, the researchers turned to something called antisense oligonucleotides.

First conceptualized more than 40 years ago, antisense oligonucleotides (ASOs) are short strings of chemically modified DNA or RNA (*oligo* in Greek means "few," and nucleotides are the structural units that make up DNA and RNA). ASOs are designed to home in on the RNA strands produced by a problematic gene and alter the gene's expression. That is, the ASOs bind to a section of the targeted RNA to produce (or, in some cases, stop the production of) proteins whose absence (or presence) causes an ailment. For decades scientists had labored to prove that this strategy could yield a drug capable of treating or preventing disease, but they found such serious problems with toxicity and delivery that many abandoned it. Yet the few researchers who pushed on overcame the obstacles just in time to benefit from the detailed information about genetic diseases revealed by the genomics revolution. "Antisense is tailor-made for diseases that have a genetic cause," says Brett Monia, who took over as CEO of Ionis in January from founder Stanley Crooke. "It's the epitome of precision medicine."

Krainer, Bennett and their colleagues called their SMA drug nusinersen. When injected into cerebrospinal fluid, it coaxes the inactive motor neuron gene to make SMN. With Biogen, they began testing the drug in human clinical trials in 2011. The Larsons enrolled Emma the day she was eligible: her second birthday. By then she could no longer crawl at all. Her first dose, in March 2015, was followed by two more doses in quick succession.

In May 2015 Dianne was in her bedroom while Emma was in the den nearby. "I hear her calling me, and it's getting closer and closer," Dianne remembers. "Next thing you know she'd crawled from the den all the way to my bedroom." Dianne asked herself, "Did I just see this?" She picked her daughter up and carried her back down the hall. Then she returned to the bedroom and called, "Emma, come here." The little girl crawled into her mother's arms. Weeping, Dianne thought, "We're on to something here!"

Indeed, they were. The clinical trial for nusinersen proved so successful that it ended a year early. The U.S. Food and Drug Administration approved the drug, under the brand name Spinraza, in December 2016. More than 8,400 patients in 40 countries are now taking it. Twenty-five newborns with the most severe SMA mutation were given the drug at birth. They are four years old now—and developing normally. "If I had done nothing else but develop Spinraza, it would have been enough," Crooke says.

But Spinraza is also exhibit A in support of the argument that ASOs are finally achieving their full potential. It is the first ASO to boast such dramatic results and commercial success. The drug earned Krainer and Bennett the multimillion-dollar 2019 Breakthrough Prize. It also put in reach a tantalizing set of neurological targets such as Huntington's disease and amyotrophic lateral sclerosis (ALS). "We discovered the genetic basis for most of these diseases back in the 1990s," Bennett says. "It's taken us 25 years to translate these really important scientific discoveries into potential therapeutics. [With Spinraza,] it was breathtaking almost to realize that we had a technology that could have such a broad impact on patients who have no therapies available to them."

Like long-distance runners who have been training at altitude, antisense scientists have put in hard miles to optimize the chemistry and delivery of oligonucleotides. Now they are at sea level and sprinting. More than 100 drugs are in the development pipeline for everything from Alzheimer's disease to hypertension. Not all will reach the finish line, but, including Spinraza, eight have been approved so far in the U.S. and Europe, all for rare diseases. Drugs for Huntington's and ALS are in the final stages of clinical trials. In a historic first, a doctor at Boston Children's Hospital created a custom antisense drug for one little girl with an ultrarare disease in less than a year. "People have been talking about biologic therapies for 30 years, and what's extraordinary is it's starting to happen," says neurologist Robert Brown of the University of Massachusetts Medical School, who is a leader in ALS research. (Biologic drugs are those made from living organisms.) "This is a true game changer."

Sense and Antisense

DNA provides the basic blueprint for life, but it has to be read and translated into action through the production of proteins, which carry out most of the work in the body. Because the instructions encoded in DNA are so critical, the process of translation has protective mechanisms built into it. There is a lot of repetition, beginning with the two strands of nucleotides that zip together to form DNA's double helix. One serves as a template, laying down sequences of the four bases that make up DNA molecules: adenine (A), thymine (T), guanine (G) and cytosine (C). The other strand reads that template and lays down a complementary set of bases. Each base on a strand is always positioned opposite its specific partner: A always pairs with T, and C with G. To ensure accuracy, the RNA only ever encodes the instructions in the nontemplate strand for the creation of proteins. Biologists call the two strands by a variety of names, including sense and antisense, which gives the ASO technology its name.

Occasionally the end results—the proteins—do not come out right. They can be overproduced or underproduced, resulting in disease. Small-molecule drugs, which make up the majority of pharmaceuticals on the market, target the proteins associated with diseases. Monoclonal antibodies, the other major class of drugs, generally bind to proteins and stimulate a patient's immune system to attack them. In contrast, the aim with antisense drugs is to disrupt the process earlier. They are designed to replace faulty RNA during the transcription process by snapping into place according to the standard base-pairing rules and thereby tweaking protein production.

A parallel effort has focused on what is known as RNA interference, or RNAi. This technology was discovered just when antisense had been given up for dead, so its proponents avoided the term, but the drugs derived from the two approaches are related. "I think of antisense as the genus and RNAi as a species," Bennett says. The difference is that RNAi drugs have two strands, whereas ASOs have only one. But any chain that is short—usually 15 to 20 nucleotides—is considered an oligonucleotide.

The versatility of oligonucleotide drug technology derives from the way it separates two critical elements: the platform or molecular properties that determine drug delivery and distribution into tissues, and the sequence of bases necessary to target a specific gene. Different sequences of bases make the information contained in the drugs distinct, but antisense drugs with the same chemical modifications tend to behave in similar ways in the body. "That's what allows us to move quickly once a platform is established to deliver to a tissue of interest," says Jonathan Watts, a nucleic acid chemist at the University of Massachusetts Medical School. "By shuffling the sequence of bases, we can dial in a totally different target using the information from a genome-sequencing experiment of a patient with a rare disease or from the genome databases. Being able to use that information intuitively and rationally is very powerful."

A Long-Distance Run

The idea of using genetic information to make a drug that could bind to RNA has been around since 1978. But there were a host of unanswered questions: How do you make an oligonucleotide into a drug? Why would binding to RNA produce an effect? Nonetheless, the idea was intriguing enough to Crooke that in 1989 he left his position as head of research and development for SmithKline (now GlaxoSmithKline) to establish a company dedicated to the development of antisense technology. He was joined there by his wife, Rosanne, also a pharmacologist, and by colleagues, including Bennett and Monia. (Originally called Isis, the company eventually changed its name, for obvious reasons, to Ionis Pharmaceuticals.)

A handful of other companies started up to pursue antisense around the same time, but one by one most abandoned the hunt. For a time it did seem that the problems of toxicity, off-target effects and a lack of potency might not be overcome.*

But Crooke and his colleagues doggedly solved the scientific problems one at a time. A long, high wall of patents at Ionis's headquarters near San Diego attests to their work. First they had to develop the necessary chemistry. For example, by modifying a key position (2') in ribose sugar in the RNA and DNA of ASOs, they were able to enhance the affinity of the ASOs for RNA receptors, thereby dramatically reducing the necessary dose. Other chemical modifications improved safety and tolerability. They also found that the drugs were not taken up into tissue when delivered directly into cells in culture, but Ionis scientists made the leap to testing the drugs in animals anyway. Monia, who ran drug development for Ionis, vividly remembers the moment when he looked at a chemical test he was using to measure levels of a specific RNA and saw almost no trace of it–the drug had entered cells in most tissues, and they had successfully knocked down the RNA's expression.

Time spent working on cancer did not prove all that fruitful, Bennett says. (Promising, more carefully designed experiments are in the pipeline, however.) What did work were drugs with specific targets, usually for rare diseases, for which proof of concept is easier to establish. The earliest ASOs were for diseases of the eye and, later, the liver, where uptake works particularly well. The drugs were effective, but they were ultimately not commercially viable, because better solutions came along.

The newest oligonucleotide drugs are designed to tackle rare diseases. One is Exondys 51, which targets Duchenne muscular dystrophy, a severe, progressive degenerative disease caused by mutations in the gene that produces the protein dystrophin. Annemieke Aartsma-Rus of Leiden University Medical Center in the Netherlands, who is president of the Oligonucleotide Therapeutics Society, is an expert in Duchenne and helped to develop the drug. It has been less spectacular than Spinraza, but on the strength of early results showing increased dystrophin levels, the drug received accelerated regulatory approval. The company marketing it (in which Aartsma-Rus has a stake) will need to show by 2021 that it makes a meaningful difference in how a patient functions.

The first RNAi drug, Onpattro, made by Boston-based biotech company Alnylam Pharmaceuticals, was approved in 2018 for treating a hereditary form of nerve damage. An approved Ionis ASO drug called Tegsedi treats the same thing. The focus now for all oligonucleotide therapies is delivering more drug more productively to more parts of the body. "A lot of people were in wait-and-see mode," Aartsma-Rus says. "They now see that if they don't start, they'll have missed the boat."

Hope for the Brain

For a long time antisense companies largely ignored neurological targets because oligonucleotides generally do not cross the blood-brain barrier. But Bennett thought that delivering them directly to the cerebrospinal fluid via lumbar puncture might work. He pushed a skeptical Crooke to let him try. "I had a lot of reservations, but the idea is to say yes," Crooke says. "'No' never made a drug, and 'no' never made anybody better." They started exploratory studies with a mouse model of Huntington's, an obvious candidate for ASOs because it is directly linked to a specific mutation. People with Huntington's carry a repeated sequence of a triplet of base pairs, CAG, that results in toxic levels of huntingtin protein and causes the progressive breakdown of brain cells. In mice, Bennett and his colleagues found that they could reduce levels of the mutant protein. "The mice actually improved," Bennett says.

Meanwhile Krainer was investigating SMA. Others had discovered that healthy people have two versions of a critical motor neuron gene, *SMN1* and *SMN2*, but the latter makes very little functional SMN protein. People with SMA do not have a functional *SMN1* gene, and their broken copy of *SMN2* cannot do the job itself. Stretches of DNA include both "exons," the coding sequences that are expressed (hence the "ex" in their name), and "introns," the noncoding stretches between exons. A process called RNA splicing joins the exons together and discards the introns. The *SMN2* gene had a variation that rendered it inactive by causing a particular coding chunk, exon 7, to be ignored. Krainer and Bennett surmised that an ASO could force that instruction chunk to be included. By 2008 they had shown that the ASO they had created worked in mice by fixing the splicing defect. The clinical trials in humans followed.

"This is what's called a disease-modifying therapy," Krainer says of Spinraza. "It isn't just dealing with some symptoms. It's getting at the root cause of the disease and changing its course." Early intervention is critical. A person with symptoms, such as Emma Larson, has already lost some motor neurons, which cannot be restored. But the treatment can prevent the remaining neurons from dying off and bring improvements in motor function. The success in treating infants has led to a push for newborn screening for SMA, which now occurs in 16 states. "The closer you start the treatment relative to birth or disease onset, the more you can achieve," Krainer says.

Spinraza's clinical success showed that, contrary to expectations, antisense therapy could be particularly effective against brain diseases. Neurological targets have "become the low-hanging fruit," Aartsma-Rus says. Several ASO-based therapeutics are in development for Huntington's, for example. One, known as RG6042, developed by Ionis and Roche, is in a phase 3 clinical trial. Earlier safety and tolerability studies showed that it is possible to lower levels of mutant proteins, says Scott Schobel, clinical science leader of the global Huntington's ASO program for Roche, but "what now is the clinical import of that?" The current trial should answer that question. "We would consider even a 30 percent slowing of decline a victory," Schobel says. That would amount to giving patients three to four months back out of a year while they are still functional.

Also known as Lou Gehrig's disease, ALS is more complicated because at most 10 percent of cases have a clear genetic cause that runs through families. The most common inherited form is caused by a mutation in a gene called *C9orf72*; another gene, *SOD1*, causes about 20 percent of familial cases. Those make up a fraction of all cases, but the promise of antisense has injected new hope where there was previously little. "My mood is sky-high," says ALS researcher Brown, who led the team that identified *SOD1* in 1993. Clinical trials for antisense drugs to treat both the *C9orf72* and the *SOD1* forms of the disease are underway. The drugs have proved safe and tolerable and suppress the activity of mutant proteins.

Part of what has clinicians such as Brown so excited is that antisense has also made it possible to develop drugs for individual patients. A young Iowa woman named Jaci Hermstad, who has a very rare form of ALS caused by a mutation in a gene called *FUS*, began taking a drug tailor-made for her in the summer of 2019. So far she is tolerating it well, and there have been small improvements, such as her regained ability to move her arm.

A Drug for Mila

A drug for just one person was science fiction until neurologist Timothy Yu of Boston Children's Hospital created a drug in less than a year (record time) for Mila Makovec, now nine years old. Mila has an ultrarare condition called Batten disease, which is really a family of disorders in which mutations cause buildups of proteins and lipids in cells. Children with Batten rarely survive into adolescence.

Like many people with Batten, Mila was unusually well coordinated and verbal early on. But at three, her toes started turning inward. Between four and five, she got clumsier and started losing her vision. Doctors at Children's Hospital Colorado eventually connected Mila's symptoms with one gene mutation for Batten that she carried.

But Batten requires two gene mutations. Mila's mother, Julia Vitarello, went looking for someone who could fully sequence Mila's genome to confirm the diagnosis. She and Mila's father also wanted to know whether their younger child, Azlan, was at risk. In January 2017 her plea reached Yu's wife via social media.

Yu's team did the sequencing and found the missing second mutation. It was caused by a jumping gene, or transposon, a sequence of nucleotides that replicates and moves to a spot in the genome where it does not belong. The discovery meant Azlan was safe. It also gave Yu an idea: it might be possible to create a drug for Mila. "We realized we could pull the Spinraza trick," Yu says. "But instead of using an antisense oligo to force an exon that was being ignored to be included, we were using an antisense oligo to shut down an exon that was getting in the way."

After several pharmaceutical companies demurred, Yu oversaw manufacture of the drug himself. Some of the $3 million Vitarello had raised in search of a cure went to the project (she prefers not to specify how much). Yu called the drug milasen, for the only patient who would receive it, and Mila got her first dose in January 2018. By then she was blind and having seizures 20 to 30 times a day, some lasting for several minutes. The damage already done to Mila's body cannot be repaired, but with treatment her seizures soon eased. After four or five months, they were lasting only a few seconds rather than minutes. Vitarello says that recently, with her help, Mila even walked up stairs with alternating feet.

When Yu reported Mila's story in the *New England Journal of Medicine* late in 2019, it made headlines. It also raised concerns about the cost and the ethics of developing a drug for one person. (Both Yu's institutional review board and the FDA approved milasen.) Bioethicist Sara Goldkind, a former FDA staffer, as well as a consultant on rare disease programs and an adviser on milasen, says that process is critical in such an unusual situation. Tests for safety and effectiveness must still be done, but there are also many mitigating circumstances—these are rare, deadly and rapidly progressing diseases with no treatments—that might allow the FDA to rely on a single adequate and well-controlled study instead of the two usually required. "There needs to be some flexible thinking in terms of how the regulations are applied," Goldkind says.

Crooke, who has stepped back from running Ionis day-to-day, set up a foundation to support the development of customized antisense drugs for ultrarare diseases affecting too few people to be viable commercially. Vitarello and Yu, too, hope to make personal treatments available to all children like Mila. One of the great advantages of antisense is that such individualized drugs can be created not just quickly but also relatively inexpensively, despite the considerable sums spent on Spinraza and milasen.

Emma the Flamingo

Like Mila, Emma Larson was not cured. The neurons she lost have not been replaced, and she has skeletal changes that are likely to be permanent. At the Larsons' home, there are wide expanses of uncarpeted wood floor, the better for Emma, who just turned seven, to zoom around in the wheelchair she calls her race car. She is in first grade, and her favorite part of the day is recess, when she likes to play on the slide and the seesaw.

When the wheelchair is parked, her parents carry her from room to room. She crawls around her playroom to show off her favorite toy, a Polly Pocket Mall. But with her walker and braces attached to a pair of sparkly pink sneakers, Emma can take a few steps under her own power. And in the dining room, with one hand on the table, she stands on the bench along the wall like a flamingo and cries, "Hey, look, standing with one leg!"

Life is still hard, the Larsons admit, but they no longer despair. They hope Emma can live independently. And they are thrilled that the newborns on Spinraza are doing so well. "That made my heart full," Dianne says as her eyes well up. "In some regards, it's a little late for Emma, but she helped pave the way for those little babies."

**Editor's Note (4/17/20): This paragraph has been edited after posting to remove an erroneous reference to one of the companies pursuing antisense therapy.*

Referenced

The Chemical Evolution of Oligonucleotide Therapies of Clinical Utility. Anastasia Khvorova and Jonathan K. Watts in *Nature Biotechnology*, Vol. 35, No. 3, pages 238–248; March 2017.

Antisense Oligonucleotide Therapies for Neurodegenerative Diseases. C. Frank Bennett et al. in *Annual Review of Neuroscience*, Vol. 42, pages 385–406; July 2019.

About the Author

Lydia Denworth is an award-winning science journalist and contributing editor for Scientific American. *She is author of* Friendship: The Evolution, Biology, and Extraordinary Power of Life's Fundamental Bond *(W. W. Norton, 2020) and several other books of popular science.*

Section 3: Drug Development and Delivery

3.1 A Better Pill—Internal Delivery Devices May Help Patients Take Their Medicine
By Knvul Sheikh

3.2 How Nanotech Powers Precision Medicine
By Robert Langer

3.3 Tiny, Tumbling Origami Robots Could Help with Targeted Drug Delivery
By Fionna M. D. Samuels

3.4 Hope for New Drugs Arises from the Sea
By Stephanie Stone

A Better Pill—Internal Delivery Devices May Help Patients Take Their Medicine

By Knvul Sheikh

Lack of compliance often leads to worsening chronic conditions and excess hospitalization. Studies consistently show one third to one half of all U.S. patients do not take their medicines as directed, and this ends up costing the health care system between $100 billion and $300 billion annually.

People fail to follow drug regimens for reasons as complex as the health care system itself. Drugs can remind people they are "sick" or generate new, unpleasant side effects. They can be costly or conflict with cultural beliefs about ingesting substances into the body. Following the instructions on the plastic bottle requires patience and training. Some protocols are painful to administer if it involves the type of injections needed to treat diabetes, infertility, osteoporosis and autoimmune diseases.

A new set of technologies may offer a way to reduce nonadherence by delivering medication a patient can swallow and forget about. In a study published Thursday in *Science* researchers described a capsule capable of autonomously injecting drugs into the top layers of stomach tissue. The swallowable, self-orienting, millimeter-scale applicator—or SOMA—safely delivered insulin to pigs in early experiments. "Many patients delay therapy because it requires an injection," says Giovanni Traverso, a gastroenterologist at Brigham and Women's Hospital and senior author on the study. In the case of diabetes, which affects nearly 10 percent of Americans, the use of insulin injections is often delayed by seven to eight years, he says. "Delivering these medicines orally can have a tremendous impact."

The inspiration for the SOMA pill came from two pieces of common scientific wisdom. The first is the practice of treating stomach ulcers with adrenaline injections. "We have experience injecting in the stomach area," he says, "and we also have a lot experience with the safety of those injections." That experience suggested drugs delivered into the stomach lining would make it to the rest of the body.

But the team needed to ensure that a self-injecting pill would reach the right location and orientation in the gastric cavity before it released its payload. The solution for this design problem came from nature. Leopard tortoises, despite being one of the largest species of that animal in the world, always can flip themselves upright because of the pointed tops of their shells. Traverso and his colleagues decided to mimic this structure with their SOMA design, so the capsules would consistently orient themselves and reliably inject insulin into the stomach wall.

The scientists loaded up to 1 milligram of insulin in a reservoir compressed behind a sugarcoated pill. Once the pill made its way into the stomach, it aligned itself with the bottom of the stomach wall. The humidity and liquids in the surroundings forced the pill's sugar coat to crack, releasing a seven-millimeter needle that successfully injected the drug into the stomach tissue. Insulin uptake began within a few minutes of ingestion and the researchers were able to see blood-glucose lowering effects in pigs, Traverso says. The amount of the drug circulating in the blood was very similar to levels seen after subcutaneous injections, he says. And by increasing the amount loaded into the SOMA reservoir, the researchers were also able to test sustained drug release for at least 30 hours.

Amrita Banerjee, an assistant professor of pharmacology at North Dakota State University who was not involved with the study is looking forward to implementation of the new technology. She's been wrestling with nonadherence among diabetics for years. But patches, skin-penetrating laser pulses, pressurized jets and other alternatives for needle-phobes have not gained in popularity, she says. Oral drugs are the pharmacological holy grail. They are the least invasive formulation, require no special equipment or training to deliver, remain stable for longer and are often cheaper to manufacture. "However, oral delivery of large molecules like insulin is a nightmare," she says.

Large molecules make up a class of drugs called biologics. These include vaccines, antibodies, gene therapies and protein- or peptide-based drugs. Their size typically means enzymes in the digestive system break them down before they can be absorbed into the blood. But SOMA pills open up possibilities for biologics to be directly injected into the stomach lining. "It's a very promising technology," Banerjee says.

Another team at Massachusetts Institute of Technology, which has collaborated with Traverso, has taken a somewhat different approach to addressing the issue of nonadherence. In a study published January 30 in *Nature Communications* the researchers described a pill that quickly inflates to the size of a ping-pong ball in the stomach, lasting up to a month and slowly releasing drugs for the duration. Like the self-orienting SOMA capsule, the inflatable pill was also inspired by evolutionary quirks. Scientists saw that puffer fish quickly inflated like a balloon when threatened, so they crafted a pill from two different hydrogels: one that would form an outer casing, and another that would soak up liquid and expand to 100 times its original size within 15 minutes of being ingested.

The hydrogel could administer drugs with a short half-life, Banerjee says. Its slow-release drug delivery could reduce the number of pills patients need to remember to take. And if the hydrogel pill needs to be removed, a patient simply has to drink a solution of calcium chloride, which will stop the drug delivery, shrink the gel back to its original size and allow it to be passed out of the body. In fact, the hydrogel is so easy to control, and so versatile, it can be used conceivably for long-term measurements of the digestive system such as temperature and pH monitoring of patients' medication-taking patterns and carrying mini cameras or other sensors into the body.

Other approaches to nonadherence deal with high-tech sensors—either in pills or on top of bottle caps—to track each time a patient takes a dose. The U.S. Food and Drug Administration has already approved one pill for schizophrenia and bipolar disorder. It sends a small electrical signal once swallowed to a temporary patch worn on the abdomen. The patch, in turn, relays the signal to a smartphone app, which stores a record of the doses consumed. "There are a lot of advances in drug-delivery systems that are being implemented in medicine," says Mark Prausnitz, director of the Center for Drug Design, Development and Delivery at Georgia Institute of Technology who was not involved with the research. But some issues still need to be resolved before some of these ingestible technologies become available on pharmacy shelves. Researchers need to demonstrate self-injecting capsules and inflatable pills will be safe over the long term, he says. Patients with diabetes and other chronic conditions will likely be using them for life. Also, there may be trade-offs between using sophisticated new delivery systems and their complexity, along with the cost to scale up their manufacturing.

One impetus driving the adoption of new drug-delivery technologies relates to the increasing approval of biologics—large molecules that must be injected to treat psoriasis, rheumatoid arthritis, multiple sclerosis and a variety of cancers. An alternative to routine shots is badly needed, Prausnitz says: "We absolutely need to make it easier for people to take their meds."

How Nanotech Powers Precision Medicine

By Robert Langer

When we think of medical breakthroughs, our minds often turn to new drugs and treatments. However, innovations in biomaterials and medicine delivery processes are just as revolutionary and important as they pave the way for such advances.

At the Massachusetts Institute of Technology, we are working at this interface of biotechnology and materials science. Take something like a burn. We can effectively treat someone with an antibiotic ointment. However, a severe burn may require more advanced treatment, such as building a skin cell polymer scaffold that helps a patient regenerate their skin. That is where our work comes in. And it's an example of how treatments are getting ever more personal to each patient.

One major focus for our team is developing polymers to deliver drugs continuously and at controlled rates for prolonged periods of time. In our research, we have created biomaterials and processes for everything from controlled drug release to tissue regeneration, and worked on anticancer drugs, gene therapy agents and vaccines alike.

This means a better response to some of the limitations of human body, and particularly its central nervous system. When we take a drug orally, it can wreak havoc on the body as it carries medicine throughout our system. By engineering polymers that offer smart delivery systems, we can target specific parts of the body. This limits exposure and therefore adverse effects, offering more effective and precise treatment.

A good example of this is treating brain disorders. Drugs taken orally–such as L-DOPA, a dopamine precursor used to treat Parkinson's disease, and Prozac, used to boost serotonin levels in patients with depression–can interact with neurotransmitters. These drugs have side effects because they act throughout the brain.

What we can do instead is deliver medicine through a miniaturized cannula–a thin tube used to deliver medicine–that is connected to small pumps implanted under the skin. This technique can deliver tiny doses (on order of hundreds of nanoliters) into brain regions as small as one cubic millimeter, giving us much more control over where medication is dispensed, according to an individual patient's needs. Research has demonstrated that this technology can control motor function. Down the line, it may help us treat tumors or neurological disorders such as Parkinson's disease or Alzheimer's.

Another exciting application of biomedical and technological innovation is telemedicine, or medical treatment from a distance. One example of this involves creating miniaturized wireless devices to treat chronic diseases or conditions that require frequent injections. Edible microchips could respond to wireless transmissions, and release drugs at sequential intervals into someone's body to treat diseases. In theory, one could have a "pharmacy on a chip" that could dispense multiple drugs in regular and accurate doses.

Right now, we are starting to see more funding of personalized treatments. This includes personalized cancer vaccines, which use messenger RNA to make vaccines against a person's own particular cancer. These treatments harness a patient's own cells to fight disease and foster the development of vaccines against a particular cancer, rather than a one-size-fits all approach. Almost all RNA therapies use nanoparticles for delivery, making technological development key for delivering medication at the right scale.

This treatment is part of a broader interest in immunotherapy and cellular-based therapies, where I expect innovation will occur in the next 30 years. The goal here is harnessing the immune system to more effectively treat diseases. This means working at a small scale to achieve more effective results.

That being said, the fruits of these labors do take some time. Regardless of the research and innovation at hand, clinical trials and funding can have significant and unpredictable effects on timelines for medical innovation and adoption.

This makes it even more crucial that we encourage innovation and support scientists and engineers. They need the freedom to explore, learn and create. They must feel that there are no limits to what they can do, that they are doing something important; and we need to raise the profile of innovative new technologies so that other teams of scientists can develop further treatments. Awards like the Millennium Technology Prize help facilitate this; in fact, since I received the prize for my research, some of the greatest strides in personalized medicine have been made by teams from across the globe.

For most diseases and illnesses, we're still at a stage where finding the right treatment is a process of trial and error; most patients are prescribed treatments because they have been proven to work for the majority, and if these don't work then it becomes a long and costly process of finding the one that is effective. But, as the developments in the areas above show, scientists and engineers are beginning to make great strides in making medicine more personal.

Nominations for the 2020 Millennium Technology Prize opened on April 1, 2019 and are accepted until July 31, 2019. They can be received from organizations such as universities, research institutes, academies of science and technology, companies and industries, and can be awarded to an individual or to a team of any nationality. More information is at millenniumprize.fi.

The views expressed are those of the author(s) and are not necessarily those of Scientific American.

About the Author

Robert Langer is an American chemical engineer, scientist and entrepreneur who is widely recognized and cited for his biotechnology research, especially in the fields of drug delivery systems and tissue engineering where his work has improved the lives of millions of patients globally. He has received numerous professional accolades including the Millennium Technology Prize–the world's largest technology prize–and is the youngest person to ever be elected to all three American science academies. He currently serves as one of the 10 Institute Professors at the Massachusetts Institute of Technology.

Tiny, Tumbling Origami Robots Could Help with Targeted Drug Delivery

By Fionna M. D. Samuels

A new kind of hollow, pea-sized robot can roll, flip and jump to navigate its surroundings. It can transition from dry surfaces to pools of liquid with ease, making it fully amphibious. Its ability to use different types of motion in multiple environments—while carrying a cargo—sets it apart from other wee machines, most of which can only move in a single way. The new bot's versatility also makes it uniquely adept at working its way through, over and around obstacles. One day its small size and multifunctionality might let it navigate the complex environment of a human body and deliver a targeted payload of medicine to a patient in need.

The robot's ability to overcome physical obstacles stems from a unique design: creased in an origami arrangement called a Kresling pattern and topped with a magnet. The Kresling pattern looks like a series of stacked right triangles wrapping around the robot's belly, making it resemble a ridged and slightly squashed cylinder. The ridges also give it a propellerlike shape that helps it move through liquid. "What we really wanted to see is whether we could integrate the geometric features with the foldability of the origami design to achieve effective navigation of the [robot] and also use its foldability mechanism for drug delivery," says Renee Zhao, an assistant professor of mechanical engineering at Stanford University. She and her colleagues describe the robot in a paper published on Tuesday in *Nature Communications.*

A small hole at one end offers access to the robot's hollow center, which can hold a small payload: an object or some liquid. A magnet at the other end allows the machine to be controlled wirelessly—all the operator needs is their own magnet. The kind of magnetic field the researchers used is similar to the type generated by a magnetic resonance imaging (MRI) machine, Zhao explains.

"I think one strategy would be developing this robot so that it's compatible with the MRI system," she says, in order to control it while a patient is in the imaging machine. Developing a new kind of device that could generate and manipulate the correct kind of magnetic field is also an option, Zhao adds, but it would need to incorporate medical imaging like an MRI machine does to track the robot's location within the body.

Some versions of the new robot have a second magnet on the opposite side of its soft, cylindrical structure. This makes the bot pumpable. An operator controlling the magnetic field generates a small amount of rotational force between the magnets, which squeezes the robot's thin plastic body. Doing this repeatedly can pump liquid from the robot's belly to its surroundings.

The device can do more than deliver liquid payloads. Its propellerlike shape means an operator can make it spin by applying a rotating magnetic field–and thereby push it through liquids. This spinning also generates enough suction to pull objects into the robot's hollow belly. And as it swims, the spinning motion holds the sucked-up payload inside. When the robot reaches its destination, the operator can stop the spinning, and the bot will dump out whatever it has picked up. This allows delivery of small solid payloads to targeted locations.

In theory, this process could carry liquid or solid medications directly to specific locations in a body–possibly in the digestive tract, for example. The robot was designed with materials that are soft enough to avoid tissue damage, Zhao says. Even the magnet is squishy, she points out. The team made it by embedding tiny glass beads and metal nanoparticles in pliable plastic. The researchers demonstrated that the robot can maneuver through the dry environment of an empty pig's stomach, as well as one filled with liquid. They controlled the robot's general trajectory, but there was no need to tell it how to maneuver around small obstacles: the magnetic field told it to move in a certain direction, and it rolled, tumbled or performed whatever other movement it took to take that path. If the robot encountered a larger obstacle, its operator could briefly increase the magnetic field's strength to make the bot jump.

If it ran into a deep pool of liquid, the operator could change the magnetic field so the device would swim.

This multifunctionality in such a simply designed robot surprised Siyi Xu, a postdoctoral robotics engineer at the Harvard Microrobotics Laboratory, who was not involved in the new study.* "It is very interesting to see them achieve many of these abilities into one integrated [design]," she says. Xu adds that many similar small robots only specialize in one kind of motion, be it walking, crawling, swimming or flying.

The new, more adept origami design could be like a blueprint for future tiny robots, Zhao says. That could open up more applications. "These functionalities are not limited to a specific disease or a specific application," she says. She and her lab are now considering how these robots might be made even smaller and able to travel in the bloodstream. Slightly larger bots could carry tiny cameras or forceps, which would be useful for minimally invasive medical procedures. Zhao plans to continue exploring similar devices, adding even more capabilities to these microrobots while maintaining their simplicity of design.

**Editor's Note (6/15/22): This sentence was edited after posting to clarify Siyi Xu's position at the Harvard Microrobotics Laboratory.*

About the Author)

Fionna M. D. Samuels was a 2022 AAAS Mass Media Fellow at Scientific American. *She's pursuing a Ph.D. in chemistry at Colorado State University. Follow her on Twitter @Fairy__Hedgehog.*

Hope for New Drugs Arises from the Sea

By Stephanie Stone

After completing six long rounds of chemotherapy, 75-year-old Pedro R. L. received the news he and his family had been hoping for: his chronic lymphocytic leukemia was in complete remission. But while his body was still recovering, he contracted COVID-19. He was admitted to the Quirónsalud Madrid University Hospital on January 30, 2021. Initial treatments failed, and by February 25 he had developed severe pneumonia. That's when his doctor, Pablo Guisado, recommended they try plitidepsin, a potent antiviral compound in a phase 3 clinical trial for treating hospitalized COVID patients.

Plitidepsin comes from a place few drugmakers would have predicted: the seafloor around Es Vedrá, an uninhabited rocky island off the southwestern coast of Ibiza, Spain. Back in 1988, Madrid-based pharmaceutical company PharmaMar organized an expedition to the storied site, an abrupt outcrop thought to have inspired Homer's tale in *The Odyssey* about singing sirens luring sailors to their death. While diving on a reef packed with purple corals and red sea fans, scientists pulled a comparatively uninspiring invertebrate creature from a rocky slope 36 meters deep–a translucent, pale-yellow tunicate, *Aplidium albicans*, that resembled a wad of discarded facial tissues.

The researchers were interested in tunicates because they filter-feed on plankton by continuously drawing water through their barrel-shaped bodies. Along with their food, they pull in viruses and other pathogens, so they need strong chemical defenses to fight off infectious organisms–and that makes them promising sources for medicines.

By 1990 PharmaMar had isolated a compound from the *A. albicans* specimen that was active against both cancer and virus cultures. PharmaMar pursued the cancer angle because cancer drugs tend to be more profitable than antivirals. After decades of research and testing, in 2018 Australia approved plitidepsin as a treatment for multiple myeloma.

When the COVID pandemic hit, company scientists quickly proved that plitidepsin was effective against SARS-CoV-2 in both laboratory cultures and mice, and it outperformed competing antivirals in preclinical, head-to-head trials. In 2020 PharmaMar launched a phase 1-2 clinical trial for hospitalized COVID patients that concluded in 2021. The results were dramatic: 74 percent of the patients with moderate disease recovered fully within a week of their first dose. The phase 3 trial is due to finish by December. In May, PharmaMar's medical director of virology Jose Jimeno said plitidepsin appeared to be superior to other COVID antivirals.* Its impact on Pedro R. L. was impressive; after two courses of treatment, his pneumonia and the rest of his symptoms had cleared completely.

Today, worldwide, there are 21 approved drugs that were sourced from the sea, most of them isolated from invertebrates. Another tunicate, *Ecteinascidia turbinata*, which attaches to submerged mangrove roots, yielded the molecular mixture that led to Yondelis, a sarcoma and ovarian cancer drug, and Zepzelca, which targets small-cell lung cancer. A black sponge that encrusts tidal pool rocks in southern Japan, *Halichondria okadai*, produced a drug, now marketed as Halaven, to treat late-stage breast cancer. And a venom peptide from a cone snail, *Conus magus*, led to Prialt, a chronic pain drug.

Corals, sea slugs, marine worms and mollusks have also yielded promising compounds. "For the past 600 million years these invertebrates have been living in this microbial soup that's like a petri dish," says marine ecologist Drew Harvell of Cornell University, explaining their need for robust defenses. An average liter of seawater contains about one billion bacteria and 10 billion viruses. Although scientists first assumed most marine invertebrates evolved their own weapons, they have learned over the past few decades that the majority of these defensive substances are actually produced by microbes living symbiotically within the creatures' tissues. Last year, for instance, a team led by Samar Abdelrahman of the Georgia Institute of Technology tested five species of sea slugs from the Red Sea and found bacteria that produced antibacterial, antifungal and anticancer agents.

Drug discovery scientists—who for decades focused on land-based biology because it was more familiar and easier to access—now widely recognize that microbes, which dominate the ocean's biological diversity, are the most likely sources of marine-derived medicines. Of 23 new drugs currently in clinical trials, 16 are produced by microbes, and another four come from invertebrates that probably owe their resilience to symbiotic microbes. In recent years scientists have isolated thousands of promising compounds from marine microbes, the diversity of which reflects the vast variability of marine conditions. "On land, microbes dry out; they have trouble maintaining a fluid balance," Harvell says. "But the oceans are a much more permissive, welcoming environment."

Yet for most approved marine drugs, the process has taken decades, partly because of insufficient funding and partly because isolating, testing and producing large quantities of novel compounds is time-consuming. Fortunately, recent advances in genomics, chemistry and computation are enabling scientists to be more targeted and efficient in the search for lifesaving medicines from the sea.

Gene Targets

In 1989 Paul Jensen brought sediments from the Bahamian seafloor back to his lab at the Scripps Institution of Oceanography to mine them for medically useful bacteria. It wasn't easy. His first challenge was to grow marine bacteria in lab conditions that are, at best, an approximation of those in the ocean. Then, when some species grew, he had to persuade them to produce at least a few of the molecules in their arsenal, even though they weren't subject to the same stimuli they would face in their natural environment.

Despite these hurdles, Jensen eventually discovered a new species of bacteria, *Salinispora tropica*, that produced a novel cancer-killing molecule. That compound, now marketed as marizomib, has just completed a phase 3 trial as a drug for glioblastoma, the deadly brain cancer that claimed the lives of John McCain and Beau Biden. It is currently awaiting approval from the Food and Drug Administration.

Marizomib is a powerful example of the potential for marine bacteria to yield new medicines, but the process took more than three decades, motivating Jensen and others to look for better approaches.

By the early 2000s genomics had transformed their work. The first full genome sequences for marine microbes, including *S. tropica*, revealed that species that produced just a few compounds in lab cultures could usually make many more; some of them had dozens of compound-encoding gene clusters in their DNA. Within a few years metagenomics–the process of sequencing the DNA of entire communities of organisms in a sample–revealed still more hidden potential. Scientists started to find compound-encoding gene clusters in species they hadn't even cultured in the lab.

Today Jensen is also looking directly for molecules instead of the microbes that produce them. On four occasions over the past year, postdoctoral researchers on his team have waded into the seagrass beds off San Diego's Point Loma peninsula to submerge sheets of tiny, absorbent beads, called resins, that pull organic molecules out of seawater. Back in the lab, Jensen analyzes the samples for bioactive compounds–chemicals that can act on a living organism.

He already has a hit: a compound with an unusual carbon skeleton that includes a group of enzyme-reactive molecules Jensen thinks could act "as something like a warhead." This novel structure might function very differently than existing medicines do. "I think it's going to kill cells," Jensen predicts. "Now we're hoping to get a sense of what its target might be."

Next, he will need to match the compound to its producer. Enormous databases of marine microbial genomes and bioactive compounds, along with the computing power necessary to correlate them, are enabling scientists to link chemicals to genes efficiently. Katherine Duncan, a marine microbial chemist at the University of Strathclyde in Glasgow, is a pioneer of this approach, which she calls pattern-based genome mining. The technique has become possible only recently. "We just haven't had the tools to compare data sets of this size," she says.

Duncan is now using this technique to analyze dark sediment cores pulled from the ocean floor 4,000 to 4,500 meters deep off the coast of Antarctica. The early results are tantalizing: The samples include at least two new species of marine bacteria, *Pseudonocardia abyssalis* and *Pseudonocardia oceani*, that produce antimicrobial compounds. On land, members of the same genus live symbiotically with fungus-growing ants, producing antibacterial and antifungal molecules that deter pathogens from invading the ants' fungal gardens. It's not a stretch to imagine that the marine cousins could yield anti-infective drugs.

One of the greatest challenges scientists such as Duncan and Jensen face is figuring out which molecular discoveries warrant the most attention. Nadine Ziemert, a microbiologist at the University of Tübingen in Germany, has developed a tool to help researchers mine genomes in a more targeted way by looking for resistance genes. Any organism that produces a toxic molecule must have some mechanism for protecting itself from its own weapon—usually by making a modified copy of the toxin's cellular target that can resist its attack.

Ziemert's tool, called the Antibiotic Resistant Target Seeker, allows researchers to access a database of more than 10,000 bacterial genomes—or upload their own—and run a search for resistance genes related to specific cell functions. The database will become more valuable as it grows, especially as researchers accelerate their work to sequence the genomes of species from extreme, underexplored environments. Ziemert's target seeker has shown such promise that start-up company Hexagon Bio has built a similar tool to mine fungus genomes for promising compounds.

New Antibiotics

Targeted genome mining couldn't come at a better time. The COVID pandemic has highlighted the need for a deeper pool of drugs to treat emerging infectious diseases. There is also a desperate need for new drugs to treat established diseases. Many bacterial infections, including pneumonia, tuberculosis, gonorrhea, blood poisoning and various foodborne diseases, have become harder—and in some cases, impossible—to treat because of rising microbial resistance to antibiotics. Public health officials widely recognize antibiotic resistance as one of the gravest threats facing humanity.

Because almost all antibiotics come from terrestrial microbes, it seems clear that marine microbes, which are greatly understudied, hold the potential to address this crisis. University of Sydney chemist Richard Payne is particularly excited about their ability to treat tuberculosis, caused by *Mycobacterium tuberculosis*. "Over the last 10 years TB has been the greatest killer among infectious diseases," Payne says, "and with all the efforts that have gone to COVID, we've gone backward with our control of TB." An antibiotic that targets a different TB protein than past drugs is needed.

That's exactly what Payne found in a bacterium from Shinyang Beach on Jeju Island, South Korea, a horseshoe of white sand on a small peninsula best known for its ideal windsurfing and kitesurfing conditions. The compound, ohmyungsamycin A, prevents *M. tuberculosis* from properly disposing of its waste proteins, ultimately killing the cell. And when Payne created a set of chemical analogs—slightly altered, chemically synthesized molecules that could be produced in volume—one of them was so potent that it completely sterilized a lab-grown tuberculosis colony in three days. The drug has already proved effective in infected zebra fish and is moving on to trials in mice.

Finding and developing new antibiotics have largely fallen to academics in recent decades because the drugs sell at such low prices that pharmaceutical companies lack the financial incentive to pursue them. The same math applies to treatments for many neglected tropical diseases, including malaria. In 2012 Scripps chemist William Gerwick isolated a molecule called carmaphycin B from a tuft of cyanobacteria growing on a boat's mooring line in a Curaçao harbor. He chemically synthesized a set of analogs that he tested against cancer cells, a frequent first line of research.

The results were not spectacular, so Gerwick turned his attention to other projects. Recently, however, a colleague suggested that they test his analogs on malaria parasites, and this time the outcome was striking. "One of them was exquisitely reactive against malaria," Gerwick says. Moreover, it wasn't toxic to human cells.

Gerwick now has funding to explore carmaphycin B as a new antimalarial drug. Whether or not it eventually becomes an approved medicine, the discovery is a reminder about the possibilities stored in the thousands of bioactive marine compounds scientists have already identified.

Carmaphycin B is also a reminder that technological advances alone won't deliver new drugs; serendipity and a willingness to capitalize on it are often required. On the day that Gerwick's former student Joshawna Nunnery collected the cyanobacteria from the mooring line, she was supposed to be diving elsewhere. But when her lab mate and diving partner contracted dengue fever, she had to cancel those plans and resorted to snorkeling near the research station instead.

Opportunities to capitalize on such serendipity are increasing as investment in ocean exploration grows. On a recent expedition to the central Pacific Ocean's Phoenix Islands archipelago onboard the Schmidt Ocean Institute's research vessel, *Falkor*, Anna Gauthier became one of the first scientists to sample deep-sea bacteria from the islands. Gauthier, a doctoral student at Harvard University, planned to conduct immune response experiments during the expedition, so she didn't immediately freeze bacteria she pulled from the sea, which is the usual practice. Instead she started culturing the organisms onboard the ship.

The technique provided an unintended benefit: survivorship was far higher than in traditional, lab-based cultures of defrosted specimens. Eighty percent of the bacteria she grew were so different from those typically encountered by mammals that they didn't trigger an immune response from mammalian cells. The finding, though still far from leading to a medical advance, has tantalizing potential for immunotherapies and vaccines.

The promise of new lifesaving medicines, paired with rising public health crises, offers tremendous motivation for scientists such as Duncan in Glasgow. "I know people who have been on last-line antibiotics and were resistant," she says. "My grandma died from sepsis. Everyone has stories like that."

Duncan hopes those stories may change within the next decade. "The marine environment is hugely undiscovered," she marvels. The next plitidepsin is out there in the ocean. It might already be in a lab.

**Editor's Note (11/18/22): This sentence was edited after posting to correct the description of Jose Jimeno's position at PharmaMar.*

About the Author

Stephanie Stone is an award-winning science journalist and video producer who covers biodiversity, sustainability and human health. She is a co-founder of bioGraphic *magazine.*

Section 4: Science Evaluates Alternative Medicine

4.1 Drug Developers Take a Second Look at Herbal Medicines
By Brendan Borrell

4.2 Traditional Medicine from Southern Mexico Offers Help with Addiction
By Peter H. Addy, Ana Elda Maqueda

4.3 Anti-Vaxxers Are Here to Stay
By Beth S. Linas

4.4 The World Health Organization Gives the Nod to Traditional Chinese Medicine. Bad Idea
By The Editors

Drug Developers Take a Second Look at Herbal Medicines

By Brendan Borrell

The tall Fulani woman carried herself into the traditional healer's hut with the bearing of a princess. Like other members of this nomadic cow-herding tribe in southern Mali, she wore a long, flowing blue dress, painted her lips with indigo and henna, and adorned her earlobes with magnificent gold crescents. Once inside, however, the old healer watched her poise wither away. She was weak from recent childbirth, the palms of her hands were pale with anemia and her forehead was hot to the touch. The woman was so terribly exhausted that she nodded off just recounting her woes. "*Soumaya*," the healer proclaimed. Malaria.

With that folk diagnosis in hand, the two Western doctors observing her visit—Bertrand Graz of the University of Lausanne in Switzerland and Merlin Willcox of the University of Oxford—got to work. The woman signed an informed-consent form, provided her medical history, and allowed the researchers to take a prick of her blood for parasite counts and other analyses. She would be taking part in a remarkable study to measure the cure rate of an herbal tea prepared with the leaves of a canary yellow poppy. By the time of her follow-up, three days later, she was well on her way to recovery.

Although many U.S. Food and Drug Administration–approved drugs have their origins in the natural world, running a clinical trial with a traditional herbal medicine falls outside mainstream practice. The conventional approach to natural drug discovery involves isolating pure compounds from plants, fungi and bacteria, screening and optimizing promising leads in the laboratory, evaluating their safety in animals and, only then, proceeding through clinical trials in humans. Yet few would quibble with the observation that the conventional approach is broken: 95 percent of experimental drugs fail in clinical trials. After too many failures, pharmaceutical companies have largely turned away from natural products. But the alternative–testing vast libraries of synthetic compounds in tiny vials–has not fared much better.

Against this backdrop, Graz and Willcox are attempting to turn the paradigm for natural products discovery upside down: starting with human studies and only isolating active compounds later. The scientists make careful observations of patients already using a variety of traditional herbal remedies to identify the most promising one, then conduct a clinical trial of that remedy. Finally, they identify the active compound, which becomes the starting point for drug development. Their approach, called reverse pharmacology, was inspired by the efforts of Indian scientists hunting for new drugs from ancient Ayurvedic medicine. The beauty of it is that even if a manufactured drug never emerges, the researchers can advise traditional healers and the communities they serve about which herbs work and which do not. And they can carry out this research with a budget suited to the developing world because the early stages require little more than a pen and paper. Their studies of a type of poppy in Mali are exhibit A for the potential success of this approach and have inspired some unexpected players in global health to take a second look at herbal medicines.

Legacy of Failure

A number of high-profile drugs available today, including aspirin and codeine, grew out of the study of plants used by humans–ethnobotany, as it is known–yet such success stories have become vanishingly rare. The problem is that there has never been a clear path to gauge the potential of a plant before millions of dollars are invested in drug development. For its part, ethnobotany has always been more descriptive than analytic. Anthropologists might spend time with a shaman in the Amazon, documenting his or her plants and methods, but they have rarely remained in the field to evaluate the efficacy of these concoctions.

Nor has simply collecting and testing every species in sight panned out. An isolated chemical that shows promise in rats or petri dishes is not necessarily safe or effective in humans. The opposite is also true. Some plant compounds may have entirely unknown mechanisms of actions that standard lab tests might miss. One high-profile attempt at such bioprospecting came from Merck, which partnered with Costa Rica's National Biodiversity Institute in the 1990s to take stock of every palm or weevil they could find in the country's national parks and evaluate its pharmaceutical potential. The project was abandoned six years ago without a single blockbuster success. In essence, big pharma's chemists decided they preferred working with compounds they could synthesize on their own, and their lawyers, no doubt, found it easier to lay claim to them with patents. Today these companies evaluate millions of these compounds for hints of biological activity through an automated process called high-throughput screening.

Of course, identifying a biologically active compound is only the first step. In the U.S., the journey from drug discovery to regulatory approval takes 12 years and costs up to $800 million. High-profile flops, such as Sanofi-Aventis's weight-loss drug Acomplia or Pfizer's cholesterol drug Torcetrapib, both of which failed only in the final stages of costly clinical trials, have demonstrated that this model is failing for the developed world. It has had even worse consequences when it comes to neglected diseases in the developing world, where most of the population cannot afford medications that are, by and large, manufactured abroad.

The lack of effective new drugs and the prohibitive cost of existing drugs are particularly troubling where malaria is concerned. Every year this mosquito-borne parasite infects 200 million people in tropical countries, killing half a million. Malaria has evolved resistance to just about everything researchers have thrown at it. In Africa, where 85 percent of the world's malaria cases occur, the current gold standard treatments, artemisinin-combination therapies (ACTs), are subsidized and theoretically available at government clinics and village shops. Yet poor roads and the availability of other, substandard medications make the drug combination's efficacy look a lot better on paper than on the ground. In one recent survey in Mali, 87 percent of children who came down with malaria were initially treated at home, and one quarter received traditional medicines alone. Taking those factors into consideration, some researchers think traditional practices deserve a closer look. But time is running out. Traditional medicine in Africa and other regions is threatened by both modernization and intense competition from Chinese herbal manufacturers, which have outposts in far-flung villages. "If we don't study it now," Graz says, "it may well vanish in large parts of the world within a single generation."

Flower Power

The idea for reverse pharmacology evolved gradually, by trial and error, as Graz and Willcox homed in on and began testing the magical poppy from Mali. Graz is a committed defender of observational studies, in which investigators make inferences about the effect of a treatment based on observation. This type of study contrasts with randomized clinical trials, which randomly assign patients to a treatment group and a control group. Graz recognizes that a randomized controlled trial is the only way to truly tell if a drug works. Yet such trials are often conducted under unrealistic conditions and with only a subset of the patient population, he notes. Although observational studies are not experiments, by documenting and analyzing patient outcomes at clinics, they give researchers a better idea of what works in the real world.

Such a counterintuitive take is what brought Graz to Mali in December 2002. He planned to a run a type of observational trial he invented called the Retrospective Treatment Outcome study, or RTO, with the help of Drissa Diallo, director of the department of traditional medicine at Mali's National Institute of Research in Public Health. Over many months, their team visited households in which a family member had recently been sick with malaria. Graz tallied 66 plants that families said they used alone or in combination to treat the illness. "The failure rate was high," Graz notes. But there was a bright spot in the data. Of the 952 patients they tracked, 30 used tea made from the leaves of *Argemone mexicana*, a poppy native to Mexico that came to Africa in the 1800s. Everyone who took it reported complete recovery. The study was like high-throughput screening but with humans, which made a promising lead all the more significant.

Graz contacted Willcox with the news. Willcox had run several clinical trials on antimalarial herbs, with mixed results. The two had previously agreed that if Graz were to identify a plant that seemed to work in the RTO, Willcox would come down to run a cohort study, which follows a group of patients over time, and, they hoped, later a clinical trial. When Graz arrived at an Internet café in the city of Sikasso in southeastern Mali to begin his background research on the poppy, however, he made a disturbing discovery. He found a paper entitled "*Argemone mexicana* Poisoning: Autopsy Findings in Two Cases." In 1998 more than 3,000 people fell ill in Delhi, India, and more than 65 died as their bodies swelled from a buildup of lymph. They had all eaten mustard seed oil adulterated with *A. mexicana*, which contains the poison sanguinarine.

Graz and Willcox were spooked. Could their promising natural remedy for malaria kill patients instead of curing them? Many effective drugs can be deadly at the wrong dosages, yet that did not seem to be happening in Mali. The researchers tried to determine the lethal dose of the *Argemone* tea by subjecting mice to increasing amounts of it, but the mice suffered no ill effects. Eventually they determined that sanguinarine occurs only in the poppy's seeds, not the leaves that go into the healer's tea.

The researchers could now proceed with their studies with a clear conscience. And in September 2004 Willcox arrived in the Malian village of Missidougou. Chief Tiemoko Bengaly, a traditional healer whose grandfather had taught him to use *A. mexicana*, was happy to take part in a study of the plant's effectiveness. In contrast with Graz's retrospective study, which looked back in time, Willcox's prospective study would follow patients forward, allowing for more exacting observations and lab tests.

On one of the healer's mud-brick, straw-roofed buildings, Willcox installed a gleaming solar panel and a car battery to run microscopes, centrifuges and an electrocardiography machine. He cautioned Bengaly to shake out the poppy seeds before preparing the tea but otherwise allowed the healer to follow his own time-tested recipe: boiling the leaves for three hours in a black cauldron, over a wood fire. It was the height of the rainy season, and nearly 100 patients were clamoring to be examined on the first day.

Early on, Bengaly prescribed a single dose of tea for three days, but Willcox noticed that patients were not recovering. When he asked if that was normal, Bengaly said that he thought that dose was more "scientific." Puzzled and concerned, Willcox asked what the usual dose was. Bengaly did not have one. He usually gave patients dried plants and told them to drink as much as possible for about a week. Implementing this higher dose, Willcox now saw results. Parasite counts dropped from around 30,000 per microliter of blood to less than 2,000. After two weeks, 89 percent of adult patients had no fever. The poppy seemed to be working.

To prove that the plant was effective against malaria, Graz and Willcox needed to bring this unorthodox drug-discovery process full circle with a randomized controlled trial. Back in Missidougou, the researchers enrolled 301 patients with malaria in the trial. They randomly assigned patients to be treated with a standardized dose of *A. mexicana* tea or with artemisinin-combination therapy and followed them for 28 days. The study, published in 2010, found that 89 percent of patients taking the poppy recovered, compared with 95 percent of patients taking ACT. The full cost of the *A. mexicana* trial, which was paid for by the Swiss Agency for Development and Cooperation, came to $500,000. Willcox and Graz estimate that using the herbal medicine instead of ACT could yield a cost savings of 75 percent.

The evidence from this relatively early stage study is so compelling that Graz and Willcox argue that *A. mexicana* tea should be recommended in Mali and other remote regions where it can be cultivated for adults with malaria that is not life-threatening. This approach could help prevent malaria from developing resistance to modern drugs and reserve scarce medicines for the most serious cases, which can lead to brain damage or death.

Reverse pharmacology dovetails with conventional drug discovery in the next phase of the process, as scientists isolate active compounds from *A. mexicana*, improve their chemical characteristics, and test these pharmaceuticals in rodents and humans in more recognizable clinical trials. Yet in contrast with the conventional model of discovery, in which chemical leads are so plentiful that they are abandoned at the first signs of trouble, reverse pharmacology has the potential to bring leads to the table that have proved to be highly effective and safe. In fact, under the conventional model, *Argemone* would have already been shelved. That is because the poppy compound that shows the greatest antimalarial activity in vitro, berberine, failed to fight the parasite in mice and humans. Why the whole plant is so effective remains a mystery, one that Graz and Willcox hope to crack with further study.

Promise And Peril

The reverse pharmacology approach is particularly well suited to finding new drugs for acute diseases such as malaria that can be easily monitored, but it is hardly restricted to such remedies. About a decade ago in India, a consortium of universities, research institutes and pharmaceutical companies began using a reverse pharmacology approach to identify potential drugs for arthritis, diabetes and hepatitis from traditional Ayurvedic medicine. Following nationwide surveys of Ayurvedic physicians, Arvind Chopra of the Center for Rheumatic Diseases in Pune, India, and his colleagues came up with a short list of promising herbs for arthritis and began observational studies in clinics alongside animal pharmacology studies. In August 2013 they published the results of their double-blind randomized controlled trial of 440 patients in *Rheumatology*, showing that a combination of four herbal extracts performed as well as celecoxib (Pfizer's Celebrex) in reducing knee pain and improving knee function.

Meanwhile Willcox and Graz have been spreading the word about reverse pharmacology, training African scientists in several countries who would like to study herbs that boost lactation in women or improve symptoms associated with HIV infection. Last December, Graz traveled to the Pacific island group of Palau, ranked as the seventh most obese nation in the world, to identify traditional medicines that are effective against diabetes and hypertension. His RTO of 30 plants revealed that *Morinda citrifolia*, a tree in the coffee family, was associated with weight loss and that *Phaleria nisidai* was associated with lower blood glucose levels. A clinical trial of *P. nisidai* is now in the works. Success against diabetes, which afflicts tens of millions of people in the developed world, could reinvigorate the hunt for natural products by pharmaceutical companies.

Not everyone is convinced this new strategy for developing drugs is appropriate. Take, for example, Nicholas White, now at Oxford, who knows firsthand about the importance of traditional medicines. In 1979 he found an obscure article in a Chinese journal about an herb called *quinghao–Artemisia annua*–which had been used for more than 2,200 years to treat malaria. Working in the lab, he identified the active compound as artemisinin and ran it through the standard gauntlet of safety trials before progressing to successful human clinical trials in the 1990s. It was, in other words, a success under the conventional model of drug discovery, which is why he is so skeptical of reverse pharmacology. "It seems a bit naive," he observes. Making basic observations of healers is one thing, but running a clinical trial is potentially unethical. "Malaria is a life-threatening infection: Is it right to give a person a bark or a toad?" he says.

Willcox and Graz are used to hearing such challenges. During a presentation Willcox gave at a meeting of the Royal Society of Tropical Medicine and Hygiene in Liverpool, an audience member pointed out that their clinical trial would not pass muster under the guidelines followed by British ethical review boards, which require Western doctors to provide a Western standard of care. Others have suggested that all the money and effort spent on the research should have gone toward administering conventional drugs. "That money would have lasted two years, and after that, what?" Willcox demands. One reason why Diallo initiated the collaboration is because Mali already has a system of approving "improved herbal medicines" and sought to expand the list and beef up the evidence for it. A Malian ethical review board approved the study, and the National Institute of Research in Public Health is now honing a standardized *A. mexicana* syrup that can be manufactured and distributed locally.

Willcox and Graz have also found an unlikely ally in the Geneva-based Medicines for Malaria Venture. "It's been an interesting journey," admits chief science officer Timothy Wells. The only organization focused on research into malaria treatments (as opposed to vaccines), it is staffed by veterans of the pharmaceutical industry, and it funds projects that follow the conventional model of drug discovery. Several years ago it paid Novartis, GlaxoSmithKline and other drugmakers to test more than six million proprietary compounds in their libraries for antimalarial activity. They came back with 25,000 hits. The study raised the bar as to how potent a compound should be to warrant further investigation, but it has not necessarily brought researchers that much closer to a novel antimalarial agent.

When Wells saw the clinical trial data for *A. mexicana*, he was floored. "It's not as a good as ACT," he says, "but the point is that it has not been optimized." Derivatives of artemisinin, for instance, have been designed to be more soluble, and quinine drugs used today have gone through several iterations to enhance their efficacy. To move things in that direction, Medicines for Malaria Venture is now funding the next phase of the research on *A. mexicana* to identify the active compounds in the drugs and measure their metabolism in the body. The organization funded a search for active compounds in another antimalarial herb, which showed promise in a clinical trial in the Democratic Republic of Congo.

Crossing Borders

In January 2013 Willcox traveled to Missidougou to pay his respects to the family of the healer Tiemoko Bengaly, who had died the previous year. It was the week that the French military began air strikes against Islamist militants in the north, and the turmoil underscored just how important it is for Africans to have local sources of medicine. In 2010 the Global Fund to Fight AIDS, Tuberculosis and Malaria terminated $18 million in malaria grants over charges of corruption, and in 2012 the fund announced it was shuttering the Affordable Medicines Facility, which has provided subsidies to importers to help get reliable drugs into village shops.

Willcox and Graz had plans to measure the public health impact of their *A. mexicana* recommendations, but the tenuous political situation put them on hold. Willcox dared to stay in the country only for a week. One morning he looked out of the car he was riding in and saw those yellow flowers rustling in a fallow field. "It's a stopgap insurance policy," Willcox says, "something to fall back on when you haven't got anything else."

Referenced

Argemone mexicana Decoction versus Artesunate-Amodiaquine for the Management of Malaria in Mali: Policy and Public-Health Implications. Bertrand Graz et al. in *Transactions of the Royal Society of Tropical Medicine and Hygiene*, Vol. 104, No. 1, pages 33–41; January 2010.

Improved Traditional Medicines in Mali. Merlin Wilcox et al. in *Journal of Alternative and Complementary Medicine*, Vol. 18, No. 3, pages 212–220; March 2012.

About the Author

Brendan Borrell, based in New York City, writes frequently for Scientific American *and reported on herbal medicines as an Alicia Patterson fellow.*

Traditional Medicine from Southern Mexico Offers Help with Addiction

By Peter H. Addy, Ana Elda Maqueda

For hundreds of years, the Mazatec people of Oaxaca in southern Mexico have conducted rituals that combine their own ancient beliefs with those of Catholicism. Healers use herbs and other plants, incense, and chanting in order to learn the cures for illness, seek out lost objects and people, and travel to spiritual or astral dimensions. The most famous component of their rituals is the "magic" mushroom, which contains the psychedelic chemical psilocybin. Another tool in the Mazatec healing toolbox is "divine sage," *Salvia divinorum*, which is said to belong to the Virgin Mary and the leaves of which are consumed for their physical and spiritual healing powers. If the patient has prepared their body and mind properly beforehand, if patient and healer are both able to sing well enough during the ceremony, and if the Catholic Saints and indigenous spirits are amenable, a ritual involving the use of Salvia can purportedly lead to profound healing.

One of the most intriguing reasons to participate in these Salvia rituals is for the healing of substance abuse and dependence. We have traveled to Oaxaca to learn from the healers and villagers about the history of Salvia and its uses. The results of our fieldwork with the Mazatec will be published later this year. The Mazatec employ Salvia as an effective treatment for arthritis and inflammation, headaches, gastrointestinal and other problems. Oaxacan villagers also told us of Salvia helping to cure people of addictions to alcohol, inhalants, and stimulants such as cocaine. They believe that the feminine entity that inhabits the plant heals the body, teaches the patient what causes and sustains the addiction, and guides the patient on the road to recovery and a balanced life.

Scientists are beginning to uncover what may be happening during these rituals, as outlined in a recently published review paper. Salvia alters dopamine levels in ancient parts of the brain responsible for motivation, reward, and the internal sense of what is going on in our bodies. The Mazatec use Salvia as part of a larger ritual and worldview that cannot be reduced to a single pharmacological mechanism. However, by studying Salvia, we may be able to better understand the addiction process in the brain and devise new treatments for stimulant-use disorders. Western medicine has developed pharmacological treatments for the abuse of opioids, alcohol, and tobacco, but not for psychostimulant abuse. Increasing our understanding of Salvia and the brain may help us to reduce the suffering of those who abuse and are dependent upon cocaine and other stimulants.

Salvia leaves contain over a dozen unique chemicals, including salvinorin-A, which is the most potent naturally occurring psychedelic substance known. It is about 10 times more potent than psilocybin, for instance. Salvinorin A is a selective kappa opioid receptor agonist, which is unlike any other psychoactive substance. Drugs like psilocybin, LSD, and MDMA produce their psychedelic effects by activating part of the serotonin system. Salvia does not affect the serotonin system – and LSD, psilocybin, and all the rest do not affect the kappa opioid system in any way.

Salvinorin-A seems to disrupt many of the effects of cocaine and the addiction cycle. For instance, rats tend to move about more frequently when given cocaine compared to placebo. Rats given salvinorin-A and then cocaine do not display this cocaine-induced hyper-locomotion. Salvinorin-A is not a general sedative though, as rats on salvinorin-A do move about as normal in an open field. Rats trained to push a lever to give themselves cocaine will do so rather frequently when they have nothing else to do. Rats given salvinorin-A will push the cocaine lever much less frequently, but will push a lever for sugar water just as frequently as usual. Salvinorin-A does not seem to suppress movement, lever pushing, or motivation for stimuli. Instead, it seems to suppress only cocaine-related behaviors and motivation.

These anti-addiction effects are likely due to salvinorin-A's influence on kappa receptors, and how the kappa system affects dopamine. Dopamine receptors and kappa receptors act in opposite and complementary ways in order to maintain balance. The first thing a stimulant like cocaine does is hijack the brain's natural reward circuitry by increasing dopamine levels in the basal ganglia. Increased dopamine feels good. It is euphoric, and it can lead to impulsive and frequent drug use. Salvinorin-A, in contrast, reduces dopamine levels in parts of the basal ganglia. This leads to what is termed "dysphoria", the opposite of the euphoria that cocaine elicits. Dysphoria is not uncontrollable sadness, weeping, and gnashing of teeth. It is more of a dissociation from the warmth and familiarity of the body and human connections. One of my research participants said they were aware of everyone and everything in the room as if through a tunnel or a long cardboard tube. You become distanced from being a body, and you can even lose connection with the body entirely.

Another factor in salvinorin-A's anti-addiction effects is *interoception*, a term that refers to both the internal state of the body at any given time, as well as the emotional response to the body. At any given time, our bodies are giving off hundreds of signals about our muscles and skin and organs and orientation and location in space. All these signals come up into the brain where they are collected in the insular cortex, which is right next to, and connected with, the basal ganglia and is also densely packed with kappa receptors.

Over time, cocaine subtly but substantially alters one's sense of interoception. When a rat or a human impulsively takes cocaine, the insular cortex compares the internal milieu of "body before drug" with that of "body on drug," finds the "body on drug" milieu to be the more pleasurable of the two, and initiates more impulsive drug use. Later, the insula compares "body on drug" to "body after drug," again finds "body on drug" more pleasurable, and initiates compulsive drug seeking and use. Over time, cocaine causes the insular cortex to devalue what used to be rewarding stimuli. Things that used to be pleasurable are not any more. The drug becomes the only thing that is pleasurable, that leads to that dopamine release. However, the addiction process is not as simple as reducing interoceptive input to the insula. Pleasurable signals are blunted, but unpleasable signals are enhanced. Aches and pains are magnified, so that a person with a long-term substance use disorder feels bad things very clearly and frequently, and feels good things very rarely, unless it is the drug.

Human studies show salvinorin-A profoundly alters interoception. We recently published a study in which we had healthy adults inhale vaporized salvinorin-A. We found that low doses of salvinorin-A increased interoception, meaning that subjects experienced their own bodies as safe and trustworthy. In contrast, high doses of salvinorin-A increased dissociation and decreased interoception, meaning that subjects lost both the ability to sustain and control attention to body sensations as well as awareness of the connection between body sensations and emotional states. These findings are in line with a study one of us conducted showing that salvinorin-A affected perception of the body.

The Mazatec have used Salvia to treat addiction for hundreds of years as part of a cultural and religious tradition that is quite outside Western pharmacology. They cultivate the plant in secret places and collect fresh leaves the day of the ritual. Patients must maintain a strict diet, abstaining from sex, alcohol, and certain foods for several weeks. Ceremonies are held at night in complete darkness and may last three to four hours. The distinction between self and other, between the internal and external worlds, breaks down during these complex rituals. The healer mediates between the patient and the spirits, asking for health and wellness. After the ceremony, the healer prepares an amulet of plant leaves and spices for the patient to carry in order to complete the ritual. We owe it to the Mazatec people that this plant has survived until now. By the cultivation of cuttings in their homes and lands over the centuries, the Mazatec have made it possible for Western science to begin to uncover its medicinal properties. We feel that this plant, the people who live with it, have more to teach us still.

About the Authors

Peter H. Addy is an associate research scientist at the Yale University School of Medicine specializing in medical informatics and psychopharmacology research. He is also a licensed clinical psychologist specializing in substance misuse.

Ana Elda Maqueda is a writer, psychologist, neuroscientist, and pharmacology PhD candidate studying the psychopharmacology of Salvia divinorum in humans. She is the founder of Xka Pastora, a NGO that does fieldwork in Mexico researching the current uses of Salvia divinorum *among the Mazatec, and promotes the further understanding of the practices and beliefs surrounding the plant.*

Anti-Vaxxers Are Here to Stay

By Beth S. Linas

The rise of vaccine-preventable diseases hits close to home for me. I have a little boy in my life who was born at just 27 weeks, spent the first three months of his life in the neonatal intensive care unit (NICU) and has a rare disease called mast cell activation syndrome. Mast cells are master regulators of the immune system and this rare disease is caused when these cells become overactive.

Overactive mast cells can cause severe allergic reactions to triggers, including vaccines. Consequent to his disease, the two-dose measles, mumps, and rubella (MMR) vaccine was contraindicated, and he did not get vaccinated. But now, at age five, as a result of the measles outbreak in New York State, he is getting pre-medication in hopes of preventing an allergic reaction when he gets the vaccine. His parents fear a major setback from the tremendous progress made in managing his rare disease but understand that getting the measles would be far worse. Large scale vaccination campaigns are meant to protect children who can't medically be vaccinated. And today, the loopholes in the system are failing them.

We can do more, as individuals and as a nation, to help protect children like this and improve public health. And we should.

It can no longer be disputed that measles, mumps, and rubella are spreading in the United States. In addition to New York, Washington state declared a state of emergency as measles cases climbed; spectators of the Detroit Auto Show may have been exposed to rubella; and the mumps virus has infected at least seven people at a U.S. Immigration and Customs Enforcement (ICE) facility in Houston. The cause for these outbreaks is undisputed: decreased vaccination rates across the country have greatly reduced the required proportion of immunized individuals needed to achieve herd or community immunity. Unless the proportion of people vaccinated increases, thus eliminating susceptibility, the spread of these diseases will continue. (The proportion of the population that needs to be immunized against measles is about 93–95 percent.)

For a country that declared measles eliminated in 2000 as the result of what the CDC calls a "highly effective measles vaccine, a strong vaccination program that achieves high coverage in children, and a strong public health system for detecting and responding to measles cases and outbreaks," it is extremely regrettable that we're seeing a resurgence in measles, mumps and rubella.

As an infectious disease epidemiologist, I've always marveled at the miracle wrought by modern science and medicine in developing and scaling the delivery of the MMR vaccine. Vaccines have widely been considered one of the greatest medical achievements in history–and yet in 2019 the World Health Organization (WHO) declared vaccine hesitancy (the delay in acceptance or outright refusal of vaccines) as one of the top 10 threats to global health.

Many have attempted to address this public health emergency by addressing the other "side" of this phenomenon. Despite suggestions to the contrary, the medical and scientific community are clear and unambiguous: vaccines are safe, effective, and not harmful.

As I have read and listened to accounts of anti-vaxxers and to those of young people who are now fact-checking their parents' choice to not vaccinate, I have been struck by how little attention is given to how the public health and scientific communities are addressing the problem. It's our job as trained experts to speak out against those who are harming the health of our children. However, it is well documented that simply repeating scientific facts and figures rarely impacts the decision processes of those who are vaccine-hesitant.

So how can the scientific community help the U.S overcome vaccine hesitancy? Ultimately, we should focus on what works. We need communication and policy approaches to address low vaccination rates, especially as rates of vaccine exemptions rise. The narrative and specific examples below are by no means exhaustive or comprehensive, but rather an attempt at sparking discussion, and ideally subsequent action, to combat this growing public health problem:

- **Stronger policies.** While immunizations are required in most states for children to attend school, we should consider stronger policies requiring childhood vaccination, for both the safety of the child and for public health. This has precedent: since 2016, Australia has greatly improved vaccination rates through its "No Jab, No Pay" immunization policy, which withholds child benefits and enacts punitive financial measures for parents who do not vaccinate their children (parents of children with medical vaccine exemptions are not penalized). A similar policy U.S policy admittedly would be complicated to enact. For example, vaccine access and cost can be an issue for some families. In addition, such a policy could put pressure on families who receive state or federal child benefits.

- **Public Education Campaigns.** While policy change is slow and challenging, the public health community, advocates and government should work together more effectively on large-scale public education campaigns. Fear of autism and other side effects from vaccination can be traced to a now discredited and retracted 1998 paper in *The Lancet*, but it is time to reframe why and how vaccines are safe. The very successful Truth Initiative has worked to increase the nation's understanding of the dangers of tobacco use among young people. Its innovation center is dedicated to designing, building, and implementing novel Web, text, TV, and mobile campaigns about the dangers of smoking (remember the shocking ads of people speaking through electrolarynx devices?). The same must be done regarding both the health benefits of vaccination and the health risks that come with a failure to vaccinate.
- **On-The-Ground Public Health Programs.** Online campaigns can be powerful, but they must be done in conjunction with boots-on-the-ground public forums. Public health experts and advocates should consider engaging more frequently in honest dialogues–not one-sided lectures–about parents' fear of vaccines. We would do well to communicate the dangers of not vaccinating face-to-face, and also explain the broader positive impacts vaccines have on cognitive development and health later in life. For example, most people are probably aware that measles is highly contagious, but how many realize that the virus can live for up to two hours

in the air after an infected person has coughed or sneezed? Or that those infected with measles can spread it starting four days before and lasting until four days after the appearance of the illness's hallmark rash? People who understand the risks shouldn't alienate those who question vaccination but should instead openly discuss the science and data–while listening to the reasons why people have concerns.

It takes a lot of effort to keep trying to dispel scientific misunderstandings about vaccines, but we should strive to do so. Personal fears of vaccination should not automatically outweigh the decades of medical gains, reduced deaths, and improved health outcomes that vaccines have brought to our country, particularly children. In some areas of science and public health, differences of opinions can be enriching, even educational–but that's not the case with discussions about vaccination.

Decades of objective scientific research, data and medical consensus have fully demonstrated the effectiveness of vaccines. It is time for policy, education campaigns, and boots on-the-ground public health campaigns to improve vaccination rates to protect the public.

The views expressed are those of the author(s) and are not necessarily those of Scientific American.

About the Author

Beth S. Linas is an infectious disease and digital health epidemiologist with the MITRE Corporation in Washington, D.C. She has worked in both the non-profit and private sectors using data-driven and evidence-based technology solutions for preventing, monitoring, and improving public health. She completed her PhD and post-doctoral training in epidemiology at Johns Hopkins Bloomberg School of Public Health. She is committed to making science and public health easier for everyone to understand. You can follow her on Twitter @bethlinas. (The author's affiliation with The MITRE Corporation is provided for identification purposes only and is not intended to convey or imply MITRE's concurrence with, or support for, the positions, opinions or viewpoints she expresses here.)

The World Health Organization Gives the Nod to Traditional Chinese Medicine. Bad Idea

By The Editors

For more than 2,000 years Chinese healers have used herbal powders and tinctures, dust made from various animal parts and strategically placed needles to treat a host of human ailments. These are used in hundreds of nations globally, but the practice in China is perhaps the most extensive, documented and catalogued. Traditional Chinese medicine (TCM) is based on the concept of qi, a system of energy that flows along meridians in the body to maintain health.

Over the past decade proponents of TCM have worked hard to move it into the mainstream of global health care–and it appears those efforts are coming to fruition. The latest (11th) version of the World Health Organization's list known as the *International Statistical Classification of Diseases and Related Health Problems* (*ICD*) will include these remedies for the first time.

According to its own mandate, the WHO sets the norms and standards for medical treatment around the globe and articulates "ethical and evidence-based policy options." It categorizes thousands of diseases and influences how doctors treat them; how insurers cover those treatments; and what kind of research is done on which ailments. More than 100 countries rely on the document to determine their medical agendas.

To include TCM in the *ICD* is an egregious lapse in evidence-based thinking and practice. Data supporting the effectiveness of most traditional remedies are scant, at best. An extensive assessment was done in 2009 by researchers at the University of Maryland: they looked at 70 review papers evaluating TCM, including acupuncture. None of the studies proved conclusive because the data were either too paltry or did not meet testing standards.

To be sure, many widely used and experimentally validated pharmaceuticals, including aspirin, decongestants and some anticancer chemotherapies, were originally derived from plants or other natural sources. Those drugs have all gone through extensive clinical testing of safety and efficacy, however. Giving credence to treatments that have not met those standards will advance their use but will also diminish the WHO's credibility.

China has been pushing for wider global acceptance of traditional medicines, which brings in some $50 billion in annual revenue for the nation's economy. And in 2016 Margaret Chan, then the WHO director, praised China's plans to do so. But while it's a good idea to catalogue TCM and make health workers aware of treatments used by millions, their inclusion in the *ICD* recklessly equates them with medicines that have undergone clinical trials.

In China, traditional medicines are unregulated, and they frequently make people sick rather than curing them. One particularly troublesome ingredient, aristolochic acid, is commonly used in traditional remedies and has been linked to fatal kidney damage and cancers of the urinary tract.

A 2018 study in the *British Journal of Clinical Pharmacology* tested 487 Chinese products taken by sick patients and discovered 1,234 hidden ingredients, including approved and banned Western drugs, drug analogues and animal thyroid tissue. And in 2012 a team led by Megan Coghlan, then at Murdoch University of Australia, identified the DNA sequences in 15 samples of traditional medicines in the form of powders, tablets, capsules, bile flakes and herbal teas. The samples also contained plants that produce toxic chemicals and animal DNA from vulnerable or endangered species (the Asiatic black bear and saiga antelope, for example) and other creatures protected by international laws.

Thus, the proliferation of traditional medicines would have significant environmental impacts on top of the negative health effects. It would contribute to the destruction of ecosystems and increase the illegal trade of wildlife. China announced last October that it was legalizing the controlled trade of rhinoceros horn and tiger bone. (The move was postponed in November, following a global outcry.) Both are believed by practitioners to have the power to cure a range of ailments, from fever to impotence–although no study has found any beneficial outcome of ingesting either. Allowing even the controlled harvest of otherwise endangered creatures will boost illegal poaching, critics say.

Until they undergo rigorous testing for purity, efficacy, dosage and safety, the WHO should remove traditional medicines from its list. These remedies should be given the same scrutiny as other treatments before being included in standard care practices.

Section 5: Reproductive and Sexual Health

5.1 Maternal Health Care Is Disappearing in Rural America
By Dina Fine Maron

5.2 Abortion Bans Based on So-Called "Science" Are Fraudulent
By Nicole M. Baran, Gretchen Goldman, Jane Zelikova

5.3 What the Science on Gender-Affirming Care for Transgender Kids Really Shows
By Heather Boerner

5.4 What Scientists Are Learning about Women's Health from Other Female Animals
By Barbara Natterson-Horowitz

Maternal Health Care Is Disappearing in Rural America

By Dina Fine Maron

By the time the pregnant woman arrived at the nearest hospital with a maternity ward—90 minutes after leaving her home in Winfield, Ala.—she was ready to deliver her baby. She made it just in time, recalls Dan Avery, an obstetrician-gynecologist who tended to patients in rural Alabama and elsewhere until his recent retirement. Too often, he says, patients are not so lucky. Some have ended up delivering on the side of the road. Winfield, located in the northwestern part of the state, does have its own hospital—but, like many rural hospitals, it no longer offers obstetrical services, Avery says, so women in labor must travel about 60 miles to Tuscaloosa. When hospital budgets get tight, Avery explains, obstetrical wards are often one of the first things to go.

The problem has metastasized across the state and the nation. In 1980, 45 of Alabama's 54 rural counties had hospitals providing obstetrical services. Today only 16 of them offer such care, and doctors say that means many, many women need to drive an hour or more to deliver their babies or even get basic prenatal care from an ob-gyn. Too many women cannot make such a long monthly trek, so they simply do without. Others seek care from their family physicians.

Such extreme access problems lead to difficult decisions. Some women in Alabama preemptively choose caesarean section births because they fear they will not make it to the hospital in time, says Dale Quinney, executive director of the Alabama Rural Health Association. Although there have been no studies proving it, Quinney believes the access issue helps explain why his state has one of the country's highest caesarean rates—35.4 percent of its births in 2015. (The national average was 32 percent that year.) The disappearing maternal care problem is common across rural America. Only about 6 percent of the nation's ob-gyns work in rural areas, according to the latest survey numbers from the American Congress of Obstetricians and Gynecologists (ACOG). Yet 15 percent of the country's population, or 46 million people, live in rural America. As a result, fewer than half of rural women live within a 30-minute drive of the nearest hospital offering obstetric services. Only about 88 percent of women in rural towns live within a 60-minute drive, and in the most isolated areas that number is 79 percent.

Maternal mortality is also significantly higher in rural areas. *Scientific American* analyzed public mortality data from the U.S. Centers for Disease Control and Prevention, and found that in 2015 the maternal mortality rate in large central metropolitan areas was 18.2 per 100,000 live births—but in the most rural areas it was 29.4. Exactly why this happens is unclear. Underlying health conditions such as hypertension or diabetes could be factors, alongside poor prenatal care and geographic access. But the numbers are troubling, and the same trend holds true for infant mortality rates, according to the analysis of CDC figures.

New analysis from the University of Minnesota Rural Health Research Center puts the situation in dire terms: "More than two thirds of rural counties in Florida, Nevada and South Dakota have no in-county obstetrical services," says one of the study's authors, Carrie Henning-Smith, a research associate at the center. The analysis, which has not yet been published, finds that this was true from 2004 through 2014 (the latest year analyzed). That means these counties had absolutely no hospitals providing obstetrical care—forcing women to travel to other counties.

Unfortunately, family physicians are not moving in to fill these care gaps in high enough numbers. And the number of family physicians offering obstetrical services has dropped by half in recent years, although many still offer basic prenatal care: In the year 2000, 23 percent of family physicians offered obstetrics—but when they were surveyed in 2010 it was only about 10 percent.

Some women manage to cobble together a workaround. Maren Webb, who lives just outside Grand Marais, Minn. (population about 1,350) lives two hours from the nearest hospital that does planned deliveries (in Duluth, Minn.). In the five years that she lived and worked in the area before giving birth to her daughter in October, she had heard countless horror stories about women in labor in the back of ambulances on the way to Duluth or those who had to deliver in the emergency room at a local hospital. To avoid those fates she says she decided to "camp out" at her parent's house–about half an hour from the hospital in Duluth–in the days ahead of her due date. Webb and her husband ended up staying with her parents for a week before she finally went into labor. "We were thankful that we had the option," she says, but they wished they could have been at home, preparing for their newborn. Still, they were grateful she had not gone into labor early while they were still at home. Her family has a history of fast deliveries–two or three hours–she says, so she might not have made it to the hospital in time.

Searching for More Answers

To understand how the U.S. got here is not a simple task. Rural health care in general has taken a hit in the past few decades as hospitals have closed and fewer doctors have sought to practice in rural areas. Eighty rural hospitals have been shuttered nationwide since 2010, and about a third of the country's remaining rural facilities are vulnerable to closure as they continue to operate under tight margins, according to findings from the latest annual Rural Relevance Study. Half of Mississippi's rural providers operate at a loss, for example, according to the report, which was presented last week at the annual National Rural Health Association (NRHA) conference in Washington, D.C. Rural communities, however, are in desperate need of care: They tend to be poorer, older and less healthy than their urban counterparts.

But obstetrics–gynecology care is particularly vulnerable because delivering a baby is such a pricey business, accounting for more than 5 percent of hospital costs. Why is it so expensive? Unlike a hip replacement, it is hard to anticipate exactly how long it will take to deliver a baby, so the number of nurses, doctors, surgeons and anesthesiologists that must be available throughout delivery adds up. Rural Americans are also less likely to be insured, and more likely to pay for their care using Medicaid–which reimburses doctors at lower rates than private insurance, making it difficult for doctors and hospitals to recover costs and make profits. Low birth volumes make the economics of obstetrical units harder still: Rural communities are generally graying, a demographic fact that reduces the number of births and makes it difficult for hospitals to financially justify having maternity wards at all. And when those wards cannot make adequate money, it leads to their shutdown.

The problem also has a multiplier effect. "It's a quality of life issue. You don't want to be the only ob-gyn in a 150-mile radius. You'd never sleep!" Michael Kennedy, associate dean for rural health education at the University of Kansas Medical Center said at the NRHA conference.

The blueprint for addressing the situation remains obtuse at best. Some medical schools think part of the solution is to train more doctors for rural work. The University of Wisconsin School of Medicine and Public Health is launching the nation's first official obstetrics–gynecology residency program for "very rural" areas, with the first resident slated to be selected next month. "Increasing the physician workforce is important," says Ellen Hartenbach, residency program director for the school's Department of Obstetrics and Gynecology. "A large percentage of people practice in the same area after residency, so the theory behind our new training track is to get people training in the smaller communities and increase their exposure," she says. (ACOG says about half of all residents practice in the state where they trained.)

There are already other ob-gyn residency programs in rural areas, Hartenbach says, and there are rural tracks in family medicine for doctors in other specialties. But official definitions of rural often just mean "not urban," she says, and the Wisconsin residency program will make sure that communities considered "very rural"–those serving fewer than 20,000 people–will be the focus. "You would be hard-pressed to find that elsewhere," she says.

Yet this is only one program, with only one resident expected for 2017. Rural health care advocates are also pushing for policy action to help fuel further changes and to incentivize work in rural America. The Improving Access to Maternity Care Act, which has already passed the House but has not yet been introduced in the Senate, would require further data collection by the Department of Health and Human Services about which geographical areas need these maternity care professionals and provide student loan forgiveness for ob-gyn work there—a benefit that is currently offered for dentists and primary care physicians in some underserved communities.

Telemedicine—offering online video call access to patients—for prenatal care could also be part of the solution, rural health experts say. But a lack of broadband internet access continues to keep that from becoming a reality in many rural areas in Alabama, says Hillary Beard, a legislative assistant for Rep. Terri Sewell (D–Ala.). "I don't think this is unique to Alabama," she says. "This is a problem for many rural areas." And too often, she says, people in Sewell's district report that they had to deliver on the side of the road because they could not make it to the hospital in time, she says.

Changing state laws to let certified nurse–midwives and nurse practitioners perform more clinical tasks might help, too, Henning-Smith says. But other cultural changes may be needed to really lure more clinicians to move to rural areas, she adds. One analysis she conducted found that rural areas—at least in the state she studied, Wisconsin—were less likely to offer child care services than their urban counterparts. That matters, of course, for working parents and their quality of life.

Yet, despite these widespread ob-gyn shortages, there is still little hard data on the long-term effects of these health access gaps. "We know a lot about the closures and about the workforce challenges, but we don't really know how these things impact women and the health of their infants," says Britta Anderson, a senior research scientist at NORC's Walsh Center for Rural Health Analysis at the University of Chicago. "We need more data on if women who travel longer distances to get care suffer more negative outcomes—emotionally and physically."

Webb, the new mother from Minnesota, says knowing about this potential harm—and reducing the burden of these distances—is essential. "No one has done this research about if these distances are increasing bad outcomes," she says. The emotional burden, however, is apparent. "If the roads aren't clear and there's a blizzard, it could take a lot longer than two hours from my house—and that, too, adds to the stress," she says. "You don't want to have this extra stress when you are in labor! You want things to flow."

About the Author

Dina Fine Maron, formerly an associate editor at Scientific American, *is now a wildlife trade investigative reporter at* National Geographic.

Abortion Bans Based on So-Called "Science" Are Fraudulent

By Nicole M. Baran, Gretchen Goldman, Jane Zelikova

We are scientists, and we believe that evidence, not ideology, should inform health care decisions. The wave of anti-abortion laws across the U.S. is the latest in a long string of attempts to falsely use the language and authority of science to justify denying people their basic human rights and inflict lasting harm. Although abortion is still legal in every state, recent legislation in Alabama, Georgia, Kentucky, Louisiana, Mississippi, Missouri and Ohio threatens the future of abortion rights in the country. Scientists should, first and foremost, value evidence, and the evidence is clear: abortion bans cause harm. They make abortions less safe and especially harm historically marginalized communities.

As scientists, we are uniquely positioned to use our privilege and position in society to speak against the new abortion bans and other public policies that threaten the reproductive freedom of our nation's people. We have the knowledge to communicate the science of reproductive health care, demonstrate the harm restrictive laws will cause and hold decision makers to account.

The public officials behind these latest abortion bans exhibit breathtaking ignorance of the science of their own proposals. When asked when a woman would still be able to obtain an abortion under his near-total ban, Alabama State Senator Clyde Chambliss uttered "I'm at the limits of my medical knowledge, but until those chromosomes you were talking about combine–from male and female–that's my understanding." The lawmaker is clearly confused about the fundamentals of reproductive science, but that hasn't stopped him from authoring the most restrictive abortion law in the country–one that threatens the health of his constituents.

So-called heartbeat bills, which ban abortion as early as after six weeks of pregnancy, are not based on science. In fact, no heart yet exists in an embryo at six weeks. Yet six states and counting enacted such bills in 2019, in addition to Alabama's near-total ban. Equally unscientific "abortion reversal" laws are also gaining traction. These laws, now on the books in eight states, require doctors to tell patients receiving a medication abortion, a safe and effective way to end an early pregnancy, that it can be reversed halfway through to save their pregnancy.

Not only is this law bad science, it is actively dangerous. The idea of abortion reversal is based on a single study of six participants that was (poorly) conducted without an ethics review board. The so-called abortion reversal procedure is experimental and has neither been clinically tested nor approved by the Food and Drug Administration. Both heartbeat bills and abortion reversal laws have been opposed by leading medical groups, including the American Medical Association and the American College of Obstetricians and Gynecologists.

Our Complacency Is Complicity

As scientists, it is our job to assess the evidence, and what we know from many countries, including the U.S., is that that restrictions to reproductive health do not stop abortions but make them less safe. In addition, attempts to limit access to legal and safe abortion violate basic human rights and increase unsafe abortions. These abortion bans will cost lives–period. Existing restrictions in more than half of U.S. states already limit access to timely and affordable abortions, and these new laws would take such constraints to new heights. For example, miscarriages may be "investigated" and prosecuted under the recent law passed in Georgia. Because one in four pregnancies end in miscarriage, such scrutiny would undoubtedly target and further traumatize people already dealing with the loss of a pregnancy.

The elected officials passing these laws are not concerned with medical expertise or scientific evidence. They actively misrepresent the work of scientists, using rhetoric to deceive the public and stoke emotional outrage. These abortion bans are ideological and cynical, they are appallingly unscientific, and they are dangerous.

We need leaders who will use science to create a safer world for all, and we, as scientists and citizens, need to hold them accountable when they don't. It is time for scientists to show up and use our voices, money and positions of privilege to push back on these oppressive and harmful abortion bans.

For too long, scientists have been afraid to wade into controversies because we were taught to believe that being outspoken would chip away at our perceived public credibility. But our persistent silence has made us complicit. Anti-choice groups continue to invoke science in support of their cause. Case in point: this year the March for Life, a protest against the practice and legality of abortion, falsely claimed that science is on the side of the anti-choice movement.

In the past, as we stood on the sidelines, science was misrepresented and weaponized to harm people. We must not only face the historical legacy of that harm but also realize that the same tactics are being used today to perpetuate oppression. And we have to vow to break our silence. The time is now. We must stand in solidarity with health care workers, activists, organizers and all who fight for reproductive justice and human rights–today and every day.

Reckoning with Science's History of Harm

Unfortunately, these latest laws build upon a long history of racist and misogynistic policies that invoke science to justify the control of people's bodies and to specifically target women and members of marginalized communities. The "science" of eugenics was used to justify sterilizing women of color and disabled people for decades. The long-disproven practice of conversion therapy is still used today in an attempt to change people's sexual orientation. Even the scientific understanding of women's biological roles as mothers and nurturers continues to be twisted to defend the patriarchy, leading some to continue to argue that the subordination and domesticity of women is somehow the "natural" moral order of the world.

It is worth remembering that historically marginalized people have long suffered directly at the hands of science. The inventor of the vaginal speculum performed horrific experiments on enslaved women. A government experiment spanning decades allowed hundreds of rural African-American men with syphilis to go untreated. And the HeLa cells that revolutionized modern medicine were taken from a poor, African-American woman as she was dying of cervical cancer without her consent or any kind of compensation for her or her descendants.

It is no surprise that the modern anti-abortion agenda itself is grounded in racism and shoddy science. The long history of using science to demonize black women and justify laws that exert control over their bodies equates to institutionally sanctioned violence. Although scientific research has provided the world with much good, it has also caused harm to countless individuals, especially people of color and sexual and gender minorities. This is a truth we must confront and a history we must not repeat.

Marginalized People Will Be Disproportionately Affected by Restrictions to Reproductive Health Care

The negative effects of restricting access to safe and affordable reproductive health services will not be evenly felt. The efforts to ban access to abortion affect all people who can get pregnant, but they create additional risks for low-income women, women of color, trans men and genderqueer people, as well as victims of intimate-partner violence or sexual abuse, who are already navigating a health care system stacked against them. Long-established restrictive laws, such as waiting periods, parental-consent requirements, state-mandated counseling and conditions for hospital admitting privileges, have imposed disproportionate barriers to reproductive freedom for these groups for decades.

Marginalized people who want to end their pregnancy may feel unsafe disclosing this information or even seeking the help they need because of the stigma or the risk of violence. Women of color already face appalling maternal mortality and infant death rates. By minimizing access to safe abortions, these women and their children will be subjected to additional risks of death and injury.

None of the recent laws include provisions for emotional, community or financial support for parents and babies. Forcing people to carry unwanted pregnancies to term, especially without addressing the multifaceted challenges associated with bringing a baby into the world, will only worsen the mental and physical health disparities and socioeconomic challenges for groups already disproportionately affected by these struggles.

Access to reproductive health care is not a women's issue–it is a human rights issue. Everyone benefits when people have access to health services and when they have autonomy to start their families on their own personal timelines.

Now Is the Time to Act

What can and should scientists do? Follow the lead of groups who have been on the front lines of these issues. Women of color have been leading the movement against this latest onslaught of policies that limit access to safe reproductive health care, as well as the reproductive restrictions that came before. Ongoing organizing and legal action by these groups, especially in the American South, have helped ensure greater access to reproductive care for those living in states with barriers to abortion access. Local groups, such as SisterSong, SPARK Reproductive Justice NOW, Access Reproductive Care–Southeast and Feminist Women's Health Center, and national groups, including the American Civil Liberties Union, Planned Parenthood and NARAL Pro-Choice America, need support to continue their work in the face of new bans. We should listen to these organizers and follow their example.

You should donate money if you can, but you can also help in many other ways. You can participate in local direct actions, including marches, educational events and organizing meetings. You can also volunteer to help transport or house women who need to travel long distances for an abortion or become an abortion clinic escort or abortion doula. You can even act as a medical model and help educate health care professionals on how to provide comfortable, affirming and culturally-competent reproductive care for all people.

And men, your efforts are especially welcome. We need to know that we are not alone in this fight.

Supporting on-the-ground initiatives is critical, but we must also look within our own research programs and consider the potential negative impact of our work and the ways it may affect vulnerable people. If you are involved in any human studies, think carefully about their design to ensure that harms to vulnerable communities are minimized and work to make sure that the benefits of your research are also just and equitable. If you are in a position of gatekeeper, prioritize the funding, publication and dissemination of research that is guided by justice and equity. As an instructor in the sciences, ensure that you are providing your students with the tools to understand and evaluate scientific information but also respect and acknowledge other ways of knowing.

Use your position of authority to advocate for evidence-based sex education in your local schools and science-based decision-making from your local public officials. Do not be afraid to use your voice and your power.

The views expressed are those of the author(s) and are not necessarily those of Scientific American.

About the Authors

Nicole M. Baran is a postdoctoral fellow at Georgia Institute of Technology and a visiting scholar at Emory University. She is a behavioral neuroscientist who studies the evolution of social behavior in both birds and fish, including pair bonding, parental behaviors, mating strategies, aggression, and vocal learning. She is the executive coordinator of the 500 Women Scientists Atlanta pod. Follow her on Twitter @NMBaranPhD.

Gretchen Goldman is the research director for the Center for Science and Democracy at the Union of Concerned Scientists and air pollution exposure scientist. She holds a Ph.D. and M.S. in environmental engineering from the Georgia Institute of Technology, and a B.S. in atmospheric science from Cornell University.

Jane Zelikova is an ecologist interested in the impacts of environmental change on natural and managed ecosystems. Her interests are broad and include tropical biogeochemistry, as well as the effects of climate change on organisms big and small. She combines a strong emphasis on research with an interest in science communication and outreach, thinking about ways to expand the role of science in tackling global issues. She is the co-founder of 500 Women Scientists. Follow her on Twitter @j_zelikova..

What the Science on Gender-Affirming Care for Transgender Kids Really Shows

By Heather Boerner

For the first 40 years of their life, Texas resident Kelly Fleming spent a portion of most years in a deep depression. As an adult, Fleming—who uses they/them pronouns and who asked to use a pseudonym to protect their safety—would shave their face in the shower with the lights off so neither they nor their wife would have to confront the reality of their body.

What Fleming was experiencing, although they did not know it at the time, was gender dysphoria: the acute and chronic distress of living in a body that does not reflect one's gender and the desire to have bodily characteristics of that gender. While in therapy, Fleming discovered research linking access to gender-affirming hormone therapy with reduced depression in transgender people. They started a very low dose of estradiol, and the depression episodes became shorter, less frequent and less intense. Now they look at their body with joy.

So when Fleming sees what authorities in Texas, Alabama, Florida and other states are doing to bar transgender teens and children from receiving gender-affirming medical care, it infuriates them. And they are worried for their children, ages 12 and 14, both of whom are agender—a identity on the transgender spectrum that is neither masculine nor feminine.

"I'm just so excited to see them being able to present themselves in a way that makes them happy," Fleming says. "They are living their best life regardless of what others think, and that's a privilege that I did not get to have as a younger person."

Laws Based on "Completely Wrong" Information

Currently more than a dozen state legislatures or administrations are considering—or have already passed—laws banning health care for transgender young people. On April 20 the Florida Department of Health issued guidance to withhold such gender-affirming care. This includes social gender transitioning–acknowledging that a young person is trans, using their correct pronouns and name, and supporting their desire to live publicly as the gender of their experience rather than their sex assigned at birth. This comes nearly two months after Texas Governor Greg Abbott issued an order for the Texas Department of Family and Protective Services to investigate for child abuse parents who allow their transgender preteens and teenagers to receive medical care. Alabama recently passed SB 184, which would make it a felony to provide gender-affirming medical care to transgender minors. In Alabama, a "minor" is defined as anyone 19 or younger.

If such laws go ahead, 58,200 teens in the U.S. could lose access to or never receive gender-affirming care, according to the Williams Institute at the University of California, Los Angeles. A decade of research shows such treatment reduces depression, suicidality and other devastating consequences of trans preteens and teens being forced to undergo puberty in the sex they were assigned at birth.

The bills are based on "information that's completely wrong," says Michelle Forcier, a pediatrician and professor of pediatrics at Brown University. Forcier literally helped write the book on how to provide evidence-based gender care to young people. She is also an assistant dean of admissions at the Warren Alpert Medical School of Brown University. Those laws "are absolutely, absolutely incorrect" about the science of gender-affirming care for young people, she says. "[Inaccurate information] is there to create drama. It's there to make people take a side."

The truth is that data from more than a dozen studies of more than 30,000 transgender and gender-diverse young people consistently show that access to gender-affirming care is associated with better mental health outcomes–and that lack of access to such care is associated with higher rates of suicidality, depression and self-harming behavior. (Gender diversity refers to the extent to which a person's gendered behaviors, appearance and identities are culturally incongruent with the sex they were assigned at birth. Gender-diverse people can identify along the transgender spectrum, but not all do.) Major medical organizations, including the American Academy of Pediatrics (AAP), the American Academy of Child and Adolescent Psychiatry, the Endocrine Society, the American Medical Association, the American Psychological Association and the American Psychiatric Association, have published policy statements and guidelines on how to provide age-appropriate gender-affirming care. All of those medical societies find such care to be evidence-based and medically necessary.

AAP and Endocrine Society guidelines call for developmentally appropriate care, and that means no puberty blockers or hormones until young people are already undergoing puberty for their sex assigned at birth. For one thing, "there are no hormonal differences among prepubertal children," says Joshua Safer, executive director of the Mount Sinai Center for Transgender Medicine and Surgery in New York City and co-author of the Endocrine Society's guidelines. Those guidelines provide the option of gonadotropin-releasing hormone analogues (GnRHas), which block the release of sex hormones, once young people are already into the second of five puberty stages—marked by breast budding and pubic hair. These are offered only if a teen is not ready to make decisions about puberty. Access to gender-affirming hormones and potential access to gender-affirming surgery is available at age 16—and then, in the case of transmasculine youth, only mastectomy, also known as top surgery. The Endocrine Society does not recommend genital surgery for minors.

Before puberty, gender-affirming care is about supporting the *process* of gender development rather than directing children through a specific course of gender transition or maintenance of cisgender presentation, says Jason Rafferty, co-author of AAP's policy statement on gender-affirming care and a pediatrician and psychiatrist at Hasbro Children's Hospital in Rhode Island. "The current research suggests that, rather than predicting or preventing who a child might become, it's better to value them for who they are now—even at a young age," Rafferty says.

A Safe Environment to Explore Gender

A 2021 systematic review of 44 peer-reviewed studies found that parent connectedness, measured by a six-question scale asking about such things as how safe young people feel confiding in their guardians or how cared for they feel in the family, is associated with greater resilience among teens and young adults who are transgender or gender-diverse. Rafferty says he sees his role with regard to prepubertal children as offering a safe environment for the child to explore their gender and for parents to ask questions. "The gender-affirming approach is not some railroad of people to hormones and surgery," Safer says. "It is talking and watching and being conservative."

Only once children are older, and if the incongruence between the sex assigned to them at birth and their experienced gender has persisted, does discussion of medical transition occur. First a gender therapist has to diagnose the young person with gender dysphoria.

After a gender dysphoria diagnosis–and only if earlier conversations suggest that hormones are indicated–guidelines call for discussion of fertility, puberty suppression and hormones. Puberty-suppressing medications have been used for decades for cisgender children who start puberty early, but they are not meant to be used indefinitely. The Endocrine Society guidelines recommend a maximum of two years on GnRHa therapy to allow more time for children to form their gender identity before undergoing puberty for their sex assigned at birth, the effects of which are irreversible.

"[Puberty blockers] are part of the process of 'do no harm,'" Forcier says, referencing a popular phrase that describes the Hippocratic Oath, which many physicians recite a version of before they begin to practice.

Hormone blocker treatment may have side effects. A 2015 longitudinal observational cohort study of 34 transgender young people found that, by the time the participants were 22 years old, trans women experienced a decrease in bone mineral density. A 2020 study of puberty suppression in gender-diverse and transgender young people found that those who started puberty blockers in early puberty had lower bone mineral density *before* the start of treatment than the public at large. This suggests, the authors wrote, that GnRHa use may not be the cause of low bone mineral density for these young people. Instead they found that lack of exercise was a primary factor in low bone-mineral density, especially among transgender girls.

Other side effects of GnRHa therapy include weight gain, hot flashes and mood swings. But studies have found that these side effects–and puberty delay itself–are reversible, Safer says.

Gender-affirming hormone therapy often involves taking an androgen blocker (a chemical that blocks the release of testosterone and other androgenic hormones) and estrogen in transfeminine teens, and testosterone supplementation in transmasculine teens. Such hormones may be associated with some physiological changes for adult transgender people. For instance, transfeminine people taking estrogen see their so-called "good" cholesterol increase. By contrast, transmasculine people taking testosterone see their good cholesterol decrease. Some studies have hinted at effects on bone mineral density, but these are complicated and also depend on personal, family history, exercise, and many other factors in addition to hormones."

And while some critics point to decade-old study and older studies suggesting very few young people persist in transgender identity into late adolescence and adulthood, Forcier says the data are "misleading and not accurate." A recent review detailed methodological problems with some of these studies. New research in 17,151 people who had ever socially transitioned found that 86.9 percent persisted in their gender identity. Of the 2,242 people who reported that they reverted to living as the gender associated with the sex they were assigned at birth, just 15.9 percent said they did so because of internal factors such as questioning their experienced gender but also because of fear, mental health issues and suicide attempts. The rest reported the cause was social, economic and familial stigma and discrimination. A third reported that they ceased living openly as a trans person because doing so was "just too hard for me."

The Harms of Denying Care

Data suggest the effects of denying that care are worse than whatever side effects result from delaying sex-assigned-at-birth puberty. And medical society guidelines conclude that the benefits of gender-affirming care outweigh the risks. Without gender-affirming hormone therapy, cisgender hormones take over, forcing body changes that can be permanent and distressing.

A 2020 study of 300 gender-incongruent young people found that mental distress–including self-harm, suicidal thoughts and depression–increased as the children were made to proceed with puberty according to their assigned sex. By the time 184 older teens (with a median age of 16) reached the stage in which transgender boys began their periods and grew breasts and transgender girls' voice dropped and facial hair began to appear, 46 percent had been diagnosed with depression, 40 percent had self-harmed, 52 percent had considered suicide, and 17 percent had attempted it–rates significantly higher than those of gender-incongruent children who were a median of 13.9 years old or of cisgender kids their own age.

Conversely, access to gender-affirming hormones in adolescence appears to have a protective effect. In one study, researchers followed 104 teens and young adults for a year and asked them about their depression, anxiety and suicidality at the time they started receiving hormones or puberty blockers and again at the three-month, six-month and one-year mark. At the beginning of the study, which was published in *JAMA Network Open* in February 2022, more than half of the respondents reported moderate to severe depression, half reported moderate to severe anxiety, and 43.3 percent reported thoughts of self-harm or suicide in the past two weeks.

But when the researchers analyzed the results based on the kind of gender-affirming care the teens had received, they found that those who had access to puberty blockers or gender-affirming hormones were 60 percent less likely to experience moderate to severe depression. And those with access to the medical treatments were 73 percent less likely to contemplate self-harm or suicide.

"Delays in prescribing puberty blockers and hormones may in fact worsen mental health symptoms for trans youth," says Diana Tordoff, an epidemiology graduate student at the University of Washington and co-author of the study.

That effect may be lifelong. A 2022 study of more than 21,000 transgender adults showed that just 41 percent of adults who wanted hormone therapy received it, and just 2.3 percent had access to it in adolescence. When researchers looked at rates of suicidal thinking over the past year in these same adults, they found that access to hormone therapy in early adolescence was associated with a 60 percent reduction in suicidality in the past year and that access in late adolescence was associated with a 50 percent reduction.

For Fleming's kids in Texas, gender-affirming hormones are not currently part of the discussion; not all trans people desire hormones or surgery to feel affirmed in their gender. But Fleming is already looking at jobs in other states to protect their children's access to such care, should they change their mind. "Getting your body closer to the gender [you] identify with–that is what helps the dysphoria," Fleming says. "And not giving people the opportunity to do that, making it harder for them to do that, is what has made the suicide rate among transgender people so high. We just–trans people are just trying to survive."

IF YOU NEED HELP *If you or someone you know is struggling or having thoughts of suicide, help is available. Call the National Suicide Prevention Lifeline at 1-800-273-8255 (TALK), use the online Lifeline Chat or contact the Crisis Text Line by texting TALK to 741741.*

About the Author

Heather Boerner is a health care and science journalist based in Pittsburgh. Her work has appeared in the Daily Beast, *the* Washington Post, *the* Atlantic, *and NPR. Follow her on Twitter @HeatherBoerner.*

What Scientists Are Learning about Women's Health from Other Female Animals

By Barbara Natterson-Horowitz

Projected on the massive screen behind me onstage, a herd of giraffes rushes across a sweep of savanna. With the video set to loop, the giraffes gallop endlessly, giving me time to slowly lean across the podium and ask my audience: "Did you spot the pregnant giraffes?" I am delivering a plenary lecture at the 2019 Nobel Conference in Stockholm. The theme of that year's conference was bioinspired medicine–finding solutions in nature to human health problems–and I wanted to call attention to the connections between women and other female animals.

As a cardiologist and evolutionary biologist, I'd been posing this question about the giraffes to medical students in my courses at Harvard University and the University of California, Los Angeles, for years, so I could tell it had landed as planned. I watched the crowd scan the troop of giraffes for evidence of pregnancy–a baby bump, a lagging mother-to-be. I suspected that few, if any, of the assembled scientists and physicians had considered this question when first taking in the scene. That was precisely my point. Given the importance of female health challenges such as pregnancy to the survival of a species–including our own–shouldn't the realities of female life in the wild be more than an afterthought for doctors and biomedical researchers?

Predators pose a daily threat to survival for all prey species, and they don't give pregnant animals a pass. Even in their final, heaviest days of pregnancy, females must evade predators. To do so, they have evolved impressive physiological adaptations.

Consider a giraffe in the last weeks of her nearly 15-month gestation. She has gained hundreds of pounds–her fetus alone weighs up to 150 pounds, but the load is much heavier when you add in the placenta, extra fluid and fat. Yet pregnant giraffes appear to flee as fast as nonpregnant individuals. If they couldn't, predators would quickly target them as easy prey. That would be the end of the line for that mother, her gestating calf and ultimately the species itself.

As I publicly expressed admiration for the giraffe's gestational athleticism, I privately cringed a bit recalling how unathletic–how un-giraffe-like–I had felt as a cardiologist in the final weeks of my own pregnancies. I was the slowest doctor in the herd of physicians responding to code blue alerts for medical emergencies at the hospital. I'd become so breathless and exhausted rushing up just two flights of stairs that once, on my way to a cardiac arrest, another physician pulled me aside to express concern for my cardiac health.

I understood why they were worried. Late in pregnancy, women are at risk of developing life-threatening diseases such as preeclampsia and heart failure. Even a healthy pregnancy places significant stress on the heart. The volume of blood that is circulating expands nearly 50 percent. To deal with this increased workload, the cardiac cells and pumping chambers of the heart must grow and transform in size and shape. Cardiologists use the term "remodeling" to describe these changes, but when things go wrong, the consequences are far more serious than a misplaced sofa throwing off the feng shui. Problems with how the heart cells get remodeled during pregnancy are linked to reduced cardiac function and even heart failure soon after delivery.

Fortunately, my cardiac health turned out to be fine: the source of my shortness of breath and fatigue was the nearly 40 pounds of fetus, fluid and fat I'd packed on by the end of the third trimester. Slowing down in the last weeks of pregnancy is perfectly normal for humans–including female cardiologists who can use the elevator instead of sprinting up the stairs.

But in the wild, pregnant animals must maintain their speed and stamina to save their lives. For pregnant gazelles, zebras, and other prey species, the ability to flee swiftly protects them from predation. The animals giving chase are often also female and sometimes also pregnant. To avoid starvation, pregnant cheetahs, hyenas, and other predators need to pursue, overtake and capture fleeing prey. A species in which pregnant females can't evade predators or capture food is doomed to extinction.

I've become fascinated by how females of other species have adapted to these challenges. I now study their biology to find possible solutions to women's health issues ranging from heart failure to breast cancer. This field of research is still emerging, but already it is generating insights that could lead to lifesaving treatments for some of the most prevalent human health concerns.

Missing Females

A multispecies approach never would have occurred to me as a young professor of medicine in the 1990s. For the first 10 years of my career, I treated many forms of heart disease but always in one species—my own. Then, in 2005, I became a cardiovascular consultant to the Los Angeles Zoo. (Zoo veterinarians occasionally invite physicians to weigh in on diagnoses or assist in medical procedures, especially when the conditions are far more common in humans than in nonhuman animals.) My patient roster expanded to include great apes, bears, lions and raptors, among others. Animal health hadn't been included in my formal medical education, so the learning curve was steep. The zoo's veterinarians and the animals themselves became my teachers as I learned that most of the diseases affecting my human patients—cardiovascular disease and cancer among them—can also develop in other species.

Over the years I grew increasingly convinced that species-spanning medicine could reveal insights for my patients that traditional human-centered approaches had not. Partnering with naturalist and science writer Kathryn Bowers, I made it my mission to raise awareness about the relevance of animal health to that of humans, launching educational and professional programs, leading research teams and writing books meant to bring the fields of human medicine, veterinary science and evolutionary biology closer together. The reception to these efforts was mostly positive, but I received a surprising degree of pushback from my own field of medicine. Some physicians seemed resistant to connecting the health of their patients and other species (beyond the transmission of certain diseases from animals to humans). Maybe they took issue with the humbling notion that veterinarians could teach them about their human patients.

Human exceptionalism, I could see, was deeply entrenched in our medical traditions. People haven't always been comfortable accepting that humans are animals. It has been my experience that human health professionals reflexively assume diseases they treat in their patients are unique to our species. (They aren't.)

Anthropocentrism wasn't the only distorted worldview slowing down the progress of medical science. Biomedical research has also long focused on males to the exclusion of females. Until 1993 the National Institutes of Health didn't require the clinical trials they funded to include women—not even studies of diseases known to be more common in women than men. Mind-bogglingly, it wasn't until 2015 that the NIH mandated the inclusion of female laboratory animals in preclinical safety studies of new medical treatments. There were rationales for not including females in biomedical studies: researchers wanted to avoid the potentially confounding effects of the estrus cycle, which can introduce variations in physiology and behavior not seen in males, and they wanted to protect potentially pregnant women, and fetuses, from thalidomide-type tragedies. Yet however well intended these investigators might have been, excluding females from studies proved enormously damaging to women's health.

To address the gaps in our medical knowledge, I began to focus my species-spanning research on major challenges in women's health. The health connections between human and nonhuman females weren't hard to find. I've published studies on ovarian cancer in flamingoes, pythons, fish and humans; hosted symposia on menstrual difficulties in great apes (including us), bats and tree shrews; and collaborated with dairy veterinarians who have deep knowledge of lactation in cows to help women with common breastfeeding problems. These experiences have transformed my understanding not only of my patients but of myself as a female. I've learned when it comes to certain aspects of my health, I may have more in common with other female animals than with my husband, brother, son or the other men in my life. I call the shared bond that links human and animal females the "sisterhood of species."

Lions Get Breast Cancer

I first glimpsed the connection among female animals while examining Cookie, a geriatric lioness, at the Los Angeles Zoo in 2012. After an operation, a lion's heartbeats sound pretty much the same as those of a human who has been through the same procedure. So the clarity of the lub-dup, lub-dups streaming through the stethoscope I had pressed against Cookie's huge, furry chest reassured me. It meant the dangerous buildup of fluid we had removed from the sac around her heart hadn't returned. The pathology report on the cause of the fluid buildup wasn't back yet, however, and the veterinarians were worried that it might be metastatic breast cancer. There were two reasons for this specific concern. First, breast cancer is one of the tumors that sometimes spreads to the heart, creating inflammation and the kind of fluid buildup that had threatened Cookie's life. The other reason, the veterinarians explained, was that compared with other zoo animals, lions, jaguars, cheetahs, and other cats are especially susceptible to breast cancer.

This connection between human and animal health was personal. Breast cancer is a health concern for many women, and I was no exception. Around the time I first learned about breast cancer in cats, I was being tested for the *BRCA* mutations following several borderline breast biopsies. The *BRCA* mutations are well known to put women at increased risk of breast and ovarian cancers. To my amazement, I learned that *BRCA* mutations also put some dog breeds, including Cavalier King Charles Spaniels, and certain other carnivores at increased risk. In all my years caring for women, as well as some men, with breast cancer, I hadn't considered what other species might also be vulnerable. In fact, as I showed in a recently published study, breast cancer is a threat across nearly all mammalian lineages, with cases found in creatures ranging from kangaroos and koalas to wombats and water buffalos.

Ultimately Cookie and I were both lucky. Cookie's fluid buildup turned out not to be cancerous, and she went on to live another four years. I tested negative for *BRCA* mutations, and my biopsies did not show breast cancer. Other creatures have not fared so well. But we have learned from their misfortune.

Whales don't usually develop breast cancer—leukemia and lymphoma are the more common cetacean cancers. So when researchers found that 27 percent of the dead belugas they examined in and around the St. Lawrence Estuary near Montreal between 1983 and 1999 had died of breast cancer, their discovery raised questions.

Looking for causes, investigators quickly locked on to several aluminum smelting factories near the estuary that were spewing chemicals known to induce breast and other cancers. The scientists determined that these chemicals probably contributed to the disease not only in the whales but also in humans who lived in the area and exhibited abnormally high cancer rates themselves. Recognizing the breast cancer "epidemic" in mammals living in this urban waterway helped to alert authorities to an environmental hazard that was also threatening human health.

Like the canaries that British coal miners brought with them to detect the presence of hazardous gases in the mines, the female belugas signaled that contaminants were putting humans at risk. Today rising levels of pollution are implicated in many challenges to women's health, including cancers, infertility, premature labor, and other disorders of the female reproductive system. Nonhuman female animals living around human communities are increasingly exposed to the same pollutants as women and girls, as the lines that once separated human and animal environments become blurred. Simply stated, the health of female animals is too important to our own to ignore. All female animals—including women and girls—are now canaries for one another. Our coal mine is the planet we share.

Giraffes Avoid Heart Failure

The connection among female animals extends beyond shared vulnerabilities. Some members of the sisterhood have evolved unique physiologies to defend against disease. The remarkable biology of some female animals prevents them from falling prey to diseases that claim millions of women's lives every year. To understand how and why such unique biology evolved and how it could save women's lives, consider my new take on the evolution of the giraffe and its improbably long neck.

Rewind to 11.5 million years ago, when the common ancestors of the modern giraffe and its closest evolutionary cousin, the okapi, roamed what is now Africa. Some of those ancestors wandered toward the rain forest and present-day Congo and eventually gave rise to the okapi. Other ancestors migrated toward the savanna and gave rise to the giraffe. Those differing environments helped to produce very different necks in these two lineages. In the rain forest, okapis were able to survive and thrive with perfectly fine albeit unspectacular necks. The ancestral giraffe's environments, in contrast, lacked dense foliage for hiding. A longer neck would have permitted horizon scanning and earlier detection of predators in an open grassland setting. At the same time, getting taller may have given proto-giraffes better access to sometimes limited foliage.

A downside to having a neck that places the head more than 2.5 meters away from the heart is that this all-important muscle must work harder with each beat to push blood vertically to the brain. This greater pressure on the heart is what we call blood pressure, and in a healthy giraffe, systolic blood pressure (the pressure when the heart is contracting) can exceed 250 millimeters of mercury (mm HG), compared with 120 mm HG or less for a healthy human.

Generally the problem with high blood pressure is that when a muscle like the heart works harder, it thickens. In humans and mice, when hearts thicken this way, they develop scarlike tissue, known as fibrosis. Hearts become stiffer than normal, limiting how far or fast an individual can move. To make matters worse, high blood pressure, also known as hypertension, can damage and weaken the heart over time. In humans, it results in a condition called HFpEF (for heart failure with preserved ejection fraction, pronounced "hef-pef"), which leads to exhaustion, shortness of breath and, potentially, death. HFpEF is the leading cause of heart failure in women, responsible for tens of thousands of deaths a year in the U.S. alone.

On the wide-open savanna, such stiffening could slow an animal down, threatening its survival. Hello, lion; goodbye, giraffe. But giraffes have found a workaround. Despite having blood pressure well above the levels that would earn human patients a stern talking-to from their doctor, both male and female giraffes can gallop at lion-evading speeds, and they appear to be resistant to HFpEF. Recent genomic research hints at how giraffes are able to flout the rules that constrain shorter animals.

In the past few years Chang Liu and his colleagues at Northwestern Polytechnical University in Xi'an, China, have published high-quality genomes of giraffe, okapi and other related animals. They discovered several mutations in the giraffe genome that are not found in the other species. One of the affected genes, *FGFRL1*, is linked to high blood pressure, which can lead to heart failure in humans. Could giraffe *FGFRL1* explain the longer-necked species' resistance to diseases associated with increased blood pressure?

To find out, the scientists tested two groups of mice to see how each would respond to an infusion of a hormone that causes blood pressure to rise. The first group of mice were "wild type," meaning that all their genes, including *FGFRL1*, were mouse genes. The second group had their *FGFRL1* sequence edited with CRISPR technology to mimic a giraffe's. After 28 days of exposure to the blood pressure–raising chemical, the wild-type mice had high levels of fibrosis, a common finding in humans with heart failure caused by hypertension. The hearts of the mice with giraffe *FGFRL1*, in contrast, appeared nearly fibrosis-free. This finding suggests that giraffes may have evolved a unique ability to suppress some of the damaging fibrosis of the heart.

Giraffes also appear to have evolved mechanisms to shield against other damaging effects of hypertension, including when it occurs during pregnancy. In humans, gestational hypertension–having high blood pressure during pregnancy–is pathological. A leading cause of fetal and maternal mortality, it occurs in up to 25 percent of pregnancies worldwide and is on the rise. For pregnant giraffes, in contrast, higher blood pressure is normal, and neither mothers nor babies seem to suffer any consequences from it. I've brought together a team of veterinarians, pathologists and OB-GYNs to uncover the unique biology that protects giraffes from gestational hypertension. We are comparing the placentas of giraffe and okapi, looking for clues to the evolution of this trait.

It will take time to figure out how to use the knowledge we obtain from such studies of female animals to prevent diseases in women. The principle is clear, though: many of the greatest threats to women's health may have already been neutralized in other species. The fixes are out there, in the bodies of the animals with whom we share our planet. As ingenious as we humans may be, the natural world is even smarter. Evolution's ability to solve problems is, according to Charles Darwin himself, "immeasurably superior to man's feeble efforts."

Rachel Carson is one of my scientific heroes, not only because she launched the modern environmental movement but also because she recognized the powerful connections across species. "In nature," she wrote, "nothing stands alone." I would add that no female stands alone. Members of the sisterhood of species are linked by common ancestry and the shared challenges and joys of being a female animal.

About the Author

Barbara Natterson-Horowitz is a cardiologist and evolutionary biologist on the faculties of Harvard University and the University of California, Los Angeles. She studies evolved adaptations in female animals that could improve women's health.

Section 6: Making Healthcare Equitable

6.1 Potential Inequities in New Medical Technologies
By Eric B. Kmiec, Jonathan Marron

6.2 Inequality before Birth Contributes to Health Inequality in Adults
By Janet Currie

6.3 A Tool Doctors Use Every Day Can Perpetuate Medical Racism
By Ashley Andreou

6.4 Antifatness in the Surgical Setting
By Ashley Andreou

Potential Inequities in New Medical Technologies

By Eric B. Kmiec, Jonathan Marron

As headline-catching new technologies emerge–like tools to "edit" our DNA–researchers, doctors, patients and the general public are excited about the future of medicine and the research that informs its practice. For some, there are obvious and critical conversations taking place about the ethics of this research, including how we do it (think "CRISPR babies" in China) and the potential for edits (intentional or otherwise) that could be passed on to future generations.

These conversations are important, but they can overshadow another equally important question. Will all patients have equal access to these new technologies?

That question requires us to look back at the blemished history of medical research and health care that has resulted in some patients–based on their race, gender, income and other factors–having poorer access to health care and poorer health in general. In some cases, this is because the system neglected them. In others, because the system blatantly abused them. The question we must ask is: Will new treatments continue or even worsen deeply rooted disparities? Or will we lay the groundwork for future treatments that benefit all people equitably?

The history of medical research and health care is critical to understand here. Black Americans, for example, have been subjected to a long list of historical exploitations, producing an understandable and widespread legacy of mistrust in the health sector. These range from the appalling use of enslaved women to create modern gynecological treatments, to the now infamous Tuskegee experiments, in which scientists observed the effects of untreated syphilis in young black men, to the story of Henrietta Lacks' cancer samples being used without her knowledge.

Beyond these striking examples, too many patients have been shut out of the American health care system: those who have lacked insurance and the ability to access health care services, who are undocumented, who don't speak English fluently, who are LGBTQ, who are imprisoned, or who have faced bias (both explicit and implicit) in a system developed and run by privileged white men.

While we are both men from populations who have not faced these historical injustices in this country, these questions and concerns are central to our work. One of us (Jonathan Marron) cares for children with cancer and studies how well children and parents understand cancer genomic sequencing and similar advanced technologies. My research has shown that families of nonwhite racial/ethnic background and those with less education have less understanding of the purpose of these tools–which is likely to manifest as mistrust and disinterest in these technologies as they move into the oncology clinic.

The other author (Eric Kmiec) is working within a health care system that serves a population of patients in Delaware that mirrors the diversity of our country. This work is focused on wielding the cutting-edge tool called CRISPR to try to develop treatments that can edit the "typos" in DNA that cause disease.

So how can we develop and use these tools to build a more equitable future and make them available to all, not just to the most privileged?

The first step is to make active choices to work with those who have been abused, neglected and left behind by the health care system to build trust in new science like CRISPR and gene therapies and the treatments they ultimately may yield.

This is both moral and essential to ensuring that new technologies will work for patients who aren't just white and of European descent, the group that has historically participated in medical research. If we want to succeed in developing the promise of treatments tailored to any individual ("personalized medicine"), we need to ensure that biomedical research includes genomic data from people of all backgrounds and with the full range of genomic variation that influences when, how and if diseases occur.

To make possible a future of personalized medicine, where each patient can receive truly genomically tailored treatment, we must first understand as many genomic variations between people as possible. If we don't do this now, new breakthroughs may not work as well for patients who aren't white and of European descent. Such inequitable advances are not advances at all.

There are efforts to counter this unfortunate past, including projects like All of Us at the National Institutes of Health, but change will also require meaningful and ongoing engagement with communities who previously have been shut out from research.

This leads us to the second critical step to avoid deepening health inequities: To build trust and comfort seeking out new breakthrough treatments, we must make sure that those doing research and providing care look more like society at large.

One approach to diversifying the workforce and building understanding of new technologies is to connect a wide range of students with these new technologies. For example, with support from a National Science Foundation grant, the Gene Editing Institute team at ChristianaCare has partnered with high schools to introduce CRISPR into the curriculum and launched a training programs for CRISPR at Delaware Technical Community College. This "teach the teachers" approach has now reached 77 college instructors from North Carolina to Washington state.

This work aims both to diversify the workforce and enhance medical literacy and trust in the medical system—even for those from communities severely mistreated by it in the past. A more diverse scientific community builds trust between researchers and potential subjects and ensures that scientific advances are equitably available to—and accessed by—all, regardless of gender, skin color, finances, etc.

As we move forward with cutting-edge research, it is vital that we understand the historical context of current inequities and mistrust of the medical system. Only then can we begin to address past injustices, engage with those who have been mistreated or left behind, and ensure that future scientific advances are equitably available to all.

Together, we must set a goal of reducing disparities with new treatments. Without intentional choices to do so, we risk maintaining—or even potentially worsening—the status quo.

The views expressed are those of the author(s) and are not necessarily those of Scientific American.

About the Authors

Eric B. Kmiec, Ph.D., is the director, Gene Editing Institute, Helen F. Graham Cancer Center & Research Institute, ChristianaCare.

Jonathan Marron, MD, MPH, is a pediatric oncologist and researcher at the Dana-Farber/Boston Children's Cancer and Blood Disorders Center and a member of the teaching faculty at the Harvard Medical School Center for Bioethics.

Inequality before Birth Contributes to Health Inequality in Adults

By Janet Currie

The COVID-19 pandemic has disproportionately hurt members of minority communities in the U.S. As of April 2022, 339 Black people out of every 100,000 had died of the coronavirus, compared with 322 of every 100,000 white people. Structural racism accounts for much of this disparity. Black people are more likely to have jobs that require them to leave their homes and to commute by public transport, for example, both of which increase the chances of getting infected. They are also more likely to get grievously ill when the virus strikes. As of March 2022, the hospitalization rate for those who tested positive for SARS-CoV-2 infection was more than two times higher for Black people than for non-Hispanic white people.

One reason for this alarming ratio is that Black people have higher rates of diabetes, hypertension and asthma—ailments linked to worse outcomes after infection with the coronavirus. Decades of research show that these health conditions, usually diagnosed in adulthood, can reflect hardships experienced while in the womb. Children do not start on a level playing field at birth. Risk factors linked to maternal poverty—such as malnutrition, smoking, exposure to pollution, stress or lack of health care during pregnancy—can predispose babies to future disease. And mothers from minority communities were and are more likely to be subjected to these risks.

Today's older Black Americans—those most endangered by COVID—are more likely than not to have been born into poverty. In 1959, 55 percent of Black people in the U.S. had incomes below the poverty level, compared with fewer than 10 percent of white people. Nowadays 20 percent of Black Americans live below the poverty line, whereas the poverty rate for white Americans remains roughly the same. Despite the reduction in income inequality between these groups, ongoing racism works through circuitous routes to worsen the odds for minority infants. For example, partly because of a history of redlining (practices through which financial and other institutions made it difficult for Black families to buy homes in predominantly white areas), even better-off Black people are more likely to live in polluted areas than are poorer white people—with a corresponding impact on fetal health. Worryingly, people disadvantaged in utero are more likely to have lower earnings and educational attainments, so that the effects of poverty and discrimination can span generations.

Researchers now have hard evidence that targeted programs can improve health and reduce inequality. Expansions of public health insurance offered to women, infants and children under Medicaid and the Children's Health Insurance Program have had a tremendous effect, improving the health and well-being of a generation—with the largest impacts on Black children. And interventions after birth can often reverse much of the damage suffered prenatally. Along with other researchers, I have shown that nutrition programs for pregnant women, infants and children; home visits by nurses during pregnancy and after childbirth; high-quality child care; and income support can improve the outcomes for disadvantaged children. Such interventions came too late to help those born in the 1950s or earlier, but they have narrowed the health gaps between poor and rich children, as well as between white and Black children, in the subsequent decades.

Enormous disparities in health and vulnerability remain, however, and raise disturbing questions about how children born to poorer mothers during the current pandemic, with all its social and economic dislocations, will fare. Disturbingly, just before the pandemic hit, many of the most essential programs were being cut back. Between 2018 and 2020, more than a million children lost Medicaid coverage because of new work requirements and other regulations, and many became uninsured. Now that the COVID death toll has exposed stark inequalities in health status and their attendant risks, Americans must act urgently to reverse these setbacks and to strengthen public health systems and the social safety net, with special attention to the care of mothers, infants and children.

The Hunger Winter

Decades of careful observation and analysis have gone into uncovering the manifold ways in which the fetal environment affects the future health and prospects of a child, and much remains mysterious. It would be unethical to run experiments to measure the toll on a fetus of, say, malnutrition or pollution. But we can look for so-called natural experiments–the (sometimes horrific) events that cause variations in these factors in ways that mimic an actual experiment. The late epidemiologist David Barker argued in the 1980s that poor nutrition during pregnancy could "program" babies in the womb to develop future ailments such as obesity, heart disease and diabetes. Initial evidence for such ideas came from studies of the Dutch "Hunger Winter." In October 1944 Nazi occupiers cut off food supplies to the Netherlands, and by April 1945 mass starvation had set in. Decades later military, medical and employment records showed that adult men whose mothers were exposed to the famine while pregnant with them were twice as likely to be obese as other men and were more likely to have schizophrenia, diabetes or heart disease.

Anyone born in the Netherlands during the famine is part of a cohort that can be followed over time through a variety of records. Nowadays many researchers, including me, look for natural experiments to delineate such cohorts and thereby tease out the long-term impacts of various harms experienced in utero. We also rely heavily on the most widely available measure of newborn health: birth weight. A baby may have "low" birth weight, defined as less than 2,500 grams (about 5.5 pounds), or "very low" birth weight of less than 1,500 grams (3.3 pounds). The lower the birth weight, the higher the risk of infant death. We have made enormous progress in saving premature babies, but low-birth-weight children are still at much higher risk for complications such as brain bleeds and respiratory problems that can lead to long-term disability.

In recent years computer analysis of large-scale electronic records has made it possible to connect infant health, as measured by birth weight, to long-term outcomes not just for cohorts but also for individuals. Studies of twins or siblings, who have similar genetic and social inheritance, show that those with lower birth weight are more likely to have asthma or attention deficit hyperactivity disorder (ADHD) when they get older. Several studies also show that lower-birth-weight twins or siblings have worse scores on standardized tests. As adults, they are more likely to have lower wages, to reside in lower-income areas or to be on disability-assistance programs. In combination, cohort and sibling studies demonstrate that low birth weight is predictive of several adverse health outcomes later in life, including increased probabilities of asthma, heart disease, diabetes, obesity and some mental health conditions.

Birth weight does not capture all aspects of a child's health: a fetus gains most of its weight in the third trimester, for example, but many studies find that shocks in the first trimester are particularly harmful. I nonetheless use the measure in my studies because it is important and commonly available, having been recorded for tens of millions of babies for decades.

Significantly, low birth weight is much more common among infants born to poor and minority mothers. In 2016 13.5 percent of Black mothers had low-birth-weight babies, compared with 7.0 percent of non-Hispanic white mothers and 7.3 percent of Hispanic mothers. Among those with college educations, 9.6 percent of Black mothers had low-birth-weight babies, compared with 3.7 percent of non-Hispanic white mothers. These inequalities in health at birth reflect large differences in exposure to several factors that affect fetal health.

The Poverty Connection

As already noted, the quality of a mother's nutrition substantially influences the health of her babies. In 1962 geneticist James V. Neel hypothesized that a so-called thrifty gene had programmed humankind's hunter-gatherer ancestors to hold on to every calorie they could get and that in modern times, that tendency, combined with an abundance of high-calorie foods, led to obesity and diabetes.

Studies on laboratory animals indicate, however, that the link between starvation and disease is not genetic in origin but epigenetic, altering how certain genes are "expressed" as proteins. Prolonged calorie deprivation in a pregnant mouse, for example, prompts changes in gene expression in her offspring that predispose them to diabetes. What is more, the effect may be transmitted through generations.

Outright starvation is now rare in developed countries, but poorer mothers in the U.S. often lack a diet rich in fruits and vegetables, which contain essential micronutrients. Deficiencies in folate intake during pregnancy are linked to neural tube defects in children, for example.

At present, one of the leading causes of low birth weight in the U.S. is smoking during pregnancy. In the 1950s pregnant women were told that smoking was safe for their babies. Roughly half of all new mothers in 1960 reported smoking while pregnant. Today, thanks to public education campaigns, indoor-smoking bans and higher cigarette taxes, only about 6 percent of pregnant women say that they smoke. And 54 percent of women who smoked in the three months before they got pregnant quit for at least the duration of their pregnancy.

Possibly because going to college places women in a milieu where smoking is strongly discouraged, mothers with higher education levels are less likely to smoke. Among mothers with less than a high school education, 11.2 percent smoke, compared with fewer than 1 percent of mothers with a bachelor's degree.

Among the many harmful chemicals in cigarette smoke is carbon monoxide (CO), which restricts the amount of oxygen carried by the blood to the fetus. In addition, nicotine affects the development of blood vessels in the uterus and disrupts developing neurotransmitter systems, leading to poorer psychological outcomes. Maternal cigarette smoking during pregnancy has also been associated with epigenetic changes in the fetus, although how these alterations affect an individual in later years remains mysterious. Vaping, which has surged since 2010, delivers high doses of nicotine, and surveys show that it has been tried by almost 40 percent of high school seniors.

This rise in popularity is extremely alarming because it could have long-term implications for fetal and infant health.

Yet another significant source of harm for fetuses is pollution. Pregnant women may be exposed to thousands of toxic chemicals in the air, water, soil and sundry products at home and at work. Complicating matters, each pollutant acts in a different way. Particulates in the atmosphere are thought to cause inflammation throughout the body, which has been linked to preterm labor and, consequently, to low birth weight. Lead, ingested through water or air, crosses the placenta to accumulate in the fetus and harm brain development. In 2005 Jessica Wolpaw Reyes of Amherst College showed that the phaseout of leaded gasoline in the U.S. led to a decrease of up to 4 percent in infant mortality and low birth weight.

A fetus may also receive less oxygen if its mother inhales CO from vehicle exhaust. In a 2009 study of mothers who lived near pollution monitors, my co-workers and I found that high levels of ambient CO were correlated with reduced birth weight. Worryingly, the effects of CO from air pollution are five times greater for smokers than for nonsmokers.

Reducing pollution can have immediate benefits for pregnant women and newborns. In a 2011 study of babies born in New Jersey and Pennsylvania, Reed Walker of the University of California, Berkeley, and I focused on mothers who lived near E-ZPass electronic toll plazas before and after they began operating. We compared them with mothers who lived a little farther from the toll plazas but along the same busy roads. Both groups of mothers were exposed to traffic, but before E-ZPass, the mothers near the toll plazas were exposed to more pollution because cars idled while waiting to pay the tolls. E-ZPass greatly reduced pollution right around the toll plazas by allowing cars to drive straight through. Startlingly, the introduction of E-ZPass reduced the incidence of low birth weight by more than 10 percent in the neighborhoods nearest the toll plazas.

In another study, my collaborators and I examined birth records for 11 million newborns in five states. We found that a shocking 45 percent of mothers lived within about a mile of a site that emitted toxic chemicals such as heavy metals or organic carcinogens—a number that rose to 61 percent among Black mothers. Focusing on babies born to mothers who lived within a mile of a plant, we compared birth weights when the facility was operating with birth weights when it was closed. For additional context, we also compared babies born within a mile of a plant with babies born in a one-to-two-mile band around the plants. Both groups of mothers were likely to be similarly affected by the economics of factory openings and closings, but mothers who lived closer were more likely to have been exposed to pollution during pregnancy. We found that an operating plant increased the probability of low birth weight by 3 percent among babies whose mothers lived less than a mile from the plant.

The racial divide in pollution exposure is profound, in part because of continuing segregation in housing that makes it difficult for Black families to move out of historically Black neighborhoods. Disadvantaged communities may also lack the political power to fend off harmful development, such as a chemical plant, in their vicinity. In the E-ZPass study, roughly half of the mothers who lived next to toll plazas were Hispanic or Black, compared with only about a tenth of mothers who lived more than six miles away from a toll plaza. And in a paper published in 2020, John Voorheis of the U.S. Census Bureau, Walker and I showed that across the entire U.S., neighborhoods with higher numbers of Black residents have systematically worse air quality than other neighborhoods. Black people are also twice as likely as others to live near a Superfund hazardous waste site. For these reasons, pollution-control measures such as the Clean Air Act have greatly benefited Black people.

Fight or Flight

Stress disproportionately impacts the poor—who have chronic worries about paying bills, for example—and also harms fetuses. A stressful situation triggers the release of hormones that orchestrate a range of physical changes associated with the fight-or-flight response. Some of these hormones, including cortisol, have been linked to preterm labor, which in turn leads to low birth weight. High circulating levels of cortisol in the mother during pregnancy may damage the fetus's cortisol-regulation system, making it more vulnerable to stress. And stress can trigger behavioral responses in a mother such as increased smoking or drinking, which are also harmful to the fetus.

One revealing study indicates that fetal exposure to maternal stress can have greater negative long-term effects on mental health than stress directly experienced by a child. Petra Persson and Maya Rossin-Slater, both at Stanford University, looked at the impact of the death of a close relative. Death can bring many unwelcome changes to a family, such as reduced income, which may also influence child development. To account for such complications, the researchers used administrative data from Sweden to compare children whose mothers were affected by a death during the prenatal period with those whose mothers were affected by a death during the child's early years. They found that children affected by a death prenatally were 23 percent more likely to use medication for ADHD at ages nine to 11 and 9 percent more likely to use antidepressants in adulthood than were children whose families experienced a death a few years after their birth.

Another pathbreaking study measured levels of cortisol, an indicator of stress, during pregnancy. By age seven, children whose mothers had higher cortisol levels during pregnancy had received up to one year less schooling than their own siblings, indicating that they had been delayed in starting school. Moreover, for any given level of cortisol in the mother's blood, the negative effects were more pronounced for children born to less educated mothers. This finding suggests that although being stressed during pregnancy is damaging to the fetus, mothers with more education are better able to buffer the effects on their children–an important finding in view of the severe stress imposed by COVID on families today.

It is no surprise that disease can also harm a fetus. Douglas V. Almond of Columbia University looked at people born in the U.S. at the peak of the influenza epidemic of 1918 and found that they were 1.5 times more likely to be poor as adults than were those born just before them. In work I conducted with Almond and Mariesa Herrmann of Mathematica looking at mothers born between 1960 and 1990 in the U.S., we found that women who were born in areas where an infectious disease was raging were more likely to have diabetes when they gave birth to their own children decades later—and the effects were twice as large for Black people.

More recently, Hannes Schwandt of Northwestern University examined Danish data and found that maternal infection with ordinary seasonal influenza in the third trimester doubles the rate of premature birth and low birth weight, and infection in the second trimester leads to a 9 percent reduction in earnings and a 35 percent increase in welfare dependence once the child reaches adulthood.

Preventing Harm

Health at birth and beyond can nonetheless be improved through thoughtful interventions targeting pregnant women, babies and children and through reductions in pollution. The food safety net in the U.S. has already had tremendous success in preventing low birth weight in the babies of disadvantaged women. The rollout of the food stamp program (now called the Supplemental Nutrition Assistance Program, or SNAP) across the U.S. in the mid-1970s reduced the incidence of low birth weight by between 5 and 11 percent. In addition, children who benefited from the rollout grew up to be less likely to have metabolic syndrome—a cluster of conditions that include obesity and diabetes. Notably, women who had benefited as fetuses or young children were more likely to be economically self-sufficient.

The 1970s also saw the introduction of the Special Supplemental Nutrition Program for Women, Infants and Children, popularly known as WIC. Approximately half of eligible pregnant women in the U.S. receive nutritious food from WIC, along with nutrition counseling and improved access to medical care. Dozens of studies have shown that when women participate in WIC during pregnancy, their babies are less likely to have low birth weight. In work looking at mothers in South Carolina, Anna Chorniy of Northwestern,

Lyudmyla Ardan (Sonchak) of Susquehanna University and I were able to show that children whose mothers received WIC during pregnancy were also less likely to have ADHD and other mental health conditions that are commonly diagnosed in early childhood.

In the late 1980s and early 1990s, state and federal governments worked together to greatly expand public health insurance for pregnant women under the Medicaid program. In work with Jonathan Gruber of the Massachusetts Institute of Technology, I showed that public health insurance lowered infant mortality and improved birth weight. Today the children whose mothers became eligible for health insurance coverage of their pregnancies in that period have higher levels of college attendance, employment and earnings than the children of mothers who did not. They also have lower rates of chronic conditions and are less likely to have been hospitalized. The estimated effects are strongest for Black people, who, having lower average incomes, benefited the most from the expansions. The fact that these babies are more likely to eventually get a college education also increases the life chances of *their* children. In the U.S., an additional year of college education for the mother reduces the incidence of low birth weight in her children by 10 percent.

Even so, too many children are still born with low birth weight, especially if their mothers are Black. Significantly, targeted interventions after birth can improve their outcomes. Programs such as the Nurse-Family Partnership provide home visits by nurses to low-income women who are pregnant for the first time, many of whom are young and unmarried. The nurse visits every month during the pregnancy and for the first two years of the child's life to provide guidance about healthy behavior. The assistance reduces child abuse and adolescent crime and enhances children's academic achievement.

Providing cash payments to poor families with young children also improves both maternal health and child outcomes, suggesting that COVID relief payments will have important protective effects. In the U.S., the largest preexisting program of this type is the Earned Income Tax Credit (EITC). Studies of beneficiaries of the EITC show that children in families that received increased amounts had higher test scores in school. With financial stress being somewhat relieved, the mental health of mothers in these families also improved. In addition, quality early-childhood education programs augment future health, education and earnings and reduce crime. Head Start, the federally funded preschool program that was rolled out beginning in the 1960s, has also had substantial positive effects on health and education outcomes, especially in places with less access to alternative child care centers.

A 2018 study, especially noteworthy in light of the tragic lead poisoning in Flint, Mich., shows that even some of the negative effects of lead can be reversed. In Charlotte, N.C., lead-poisoned children who received lead remediation, nutritional and medical assessments, WIC and special training for their caregivers saw reductions in problem behaviors and advanced school performance.

Looking Ahead

Investments in pregnant women and infants have been paying off, their success reflected in dramatically falling infant mortality rates in the U.S.–despite rising inequality in income and wealth. Alarmingly, however, many successful programs, such as the Clean Air Act, SNAP and Medicaid, are under attack. The Coronavirus Aid, Relief and Economic Security (CARES) Act passed in March 2020 provided some relief, at least with respect to Medicaid. CARES temporarily suspended disenrollment from the program, giving additional flexibility to state Medicaid programs in terms of time lines and eligibility procedures. Still, states may be hard-pressed to enroll the many who will become newly eligible for Medicaid because of job loss. Moreover, states that have not expanded the Medicaid program to cover otherwise ineligible low-income adults, as allowed by the Affordable Care Act, may see many more uninsured.

A National Academies of Sciences, Engineering and Medicine report published in 2019 laid out a road map for reducing child poverty by half within 10 years. One of the most stunning findings of the report is that it is feasible to meet that target by expanding programs that already exist. Following these directions would have a profound impact on health and health disparities. Targeted approaches, such as more thorough investigation of maternal deaths occurring up to one year after a birth, are also necessary. Even simple preventive measures such as giving pregnant women flu shots can have a tremendously positive effect on infant health and child development. Diagnosis and treatment of conditions such as preeclampsia (high blood pressure associated with pregnancy) are key to both protecting babies and lowering maternal mortality rates. It is important to help pregnant women quit smoking and to develop new approaches relevant to a new generation addicted to vaping. Also needed are stronger protections for women at risk of domestic violence, which leads directly to chronic stress, premature deliveries and low birth weight.

One salient open question is what effect the pandemic will have on the generation of children affected by it in utero and in early life. COVID itself may have negative effects on the developing fetus. The latest data suggest that although the overall risk is low, pregnant women are at increased risk of becoming critically ill (as they are with influenza or SARS). Affected babies, however, do not seem to be at risk of obvious birth defects (as they are with the Zika virus). Still, given the fact that COVID affects many body systems, it may prove to have subtler negative effects on the developing fetus. The pandemic is also an extremely stressful event compounded by the sharpest economic downturn since the Great Depression. The years 2020 and 2021 saw marked increases in domestic violence, alcohol consumption and drug overdoses, all of which are known to be harmful to the developing fetus. In consequence, the generation being born now is likely to be at increased risk going forward and will require intensive social investments to overcome its poorer start in life.

In a July 2020 sermon on the late civil rights leader John Robert Lewis, Reverend James Lawson recounted the significant gains for Americans of all colors that had resulted from that movement. He went on to ask that America's political leaders "work unfalteringly on behalf of every boy and every girl, so that every baby born on these shores will have access to the tree of life ... let all the people of the U.S.A. determine that we will not be quiet as long as any child dies in the first year of life in the United States. We will not be quiet as long as the largest poverty group in our nation are women and children." As we rebuild our shattered safety nets and public health systems in the aftermath of COVID, we need to seize the moment and use the knowledge we have gained about how to protect mothers and babies–to give every child the opportunity to flourish.

About the Author

Janet Currie is Henry Putnam Professor of Economics and Public Affairs and co-director of the Center for Health and Wellbeing at Princeton University. She studies socioeconomic differences in health and access to health care, as well as environmental threats to health.

A Tool Doctors Use Every Day Can Perpetuate Medical Racism

By Ashley Andreou

COVID-19 exacerbated various preexisting racial health disparities, which ushered in a racial reckoning in the medical field. As a result, many medical institutions attempted to implement meaningful changes to dismantle systemic racism within their teaching and clinical environments. Yet, a tool used daily by almost every physician, the history of present illness (HPI), may still perpetuate medical racism.

"A 21-year-old African American female presented in the emergency department with diabetic ketoacidosis." The first line of a patient's history often includes their race. Many physicians believe race is an important aspect of clinical decision-making, useful for identifying risk factors and treatment options. However, these labels are inaccurate proxies for risk factors and treatment contraindications and can even hurt patients. In particular, these labels could reinforce racial biases and prevent patients from receiving standard medical treatments.

Physicians often determine racial and ethnic labels themselves rather than asking patients to self-identify. Providers who are not racially/ethnically concordant with their patients—that is, both come from different racial or ethnic background—may incorrectly conflate race, ethnicity and ancestry. Additionally, patients are typically asked to self-identify in clinical trials. So, when choosing patient descriptors, doctors may reinforce biases rather than exact some biological relationship identified by researchers. In reality, many patients do not even self-identify into categories used by researchers, making the entire process of categorization obsolete.

Beyond the issue of physicians using inaccurate racial labels, research has proven what scholars like W.E.B. Du Bois and Derrick Bell stated for decades: race is a social construct. In particular, a person's phenotype, how someone physically presents, may not hold meaningful clues for their genotype, someone's genetic make-up. For instance, a landmark study in the journal *Science* found that two people of European descent may be more genetically similar to an Asian person than they are to each other. Thus, even when patients self-identify, their race is not a clinically valuable identifier.

Finally, the practice is inconsistently used, where health care providers were more likely to include race in a patient's HPI if they were a Black American. This pattern by clinicians highlights how these labels are often an unwieldy outlet for bias rather than evidence-based clinical practice. In fact, when physicians focus on race it is more likely to detract from care than bolster it, negatively affecting aspects of patient care like the time allotted for a visit.

The relationship between race and certain diseases, such as diabetes, sarcoidosis and lupus, is complex or not well understood. Some doctors may argue that patients' race is needed to crystallize their differential diagnosis but, outside of race, there is a constellation of symptoms that elucidate the clinical picture of these diseases, which makes it an unnecessary addition. Physicians who ascribe race as a risk factor for diseases like diabetes, cancer and cardiovascular disease might miss a diagnosis in some cases may also misconstrue upstream, social determinants of health as innate genetic differences.

By erasing these modifiable factors (e.g., access to nutritious food, socioeconomic status, stress levels, access to health care, environmental health, etc.), which are maintained by systemic racism, the medical field unfairly places onus on a patient's genetics. This practice has the potential to fuel racial bias amongst the general public, as many people look to the medical community to understand biological minutia and operate on objectivity. By using this outdated practice, physicians may be reinforcing the incorrect idea that race differentiation holds scientific value instead of being a clumsy artifact of the profession.

Unfortunately, this practice may not only stoke racist beliefs but also introduce immediate bodily harm on Black and brown bodies. In certain medical formulas, such as estimated glomerular filtration rate (eGFR) and vaginal birth after Cesarean section

(VBAC), plugging in a Black or nonwhite Hispanic patient's race into the calculations could preclude them from receiving a kidney transplant or being offered a vaginal birth.

In addition, codifying a patient's race in their medical records may limit them from receiving high-quality treatment. Clozapine, an effective antipsychotic, is underprescribed in Black American populations because of the fear of benign ethnic neutropenia (BEN), defined as an absolute neutrophil (a type of white blood cell that aids a person's immune system) count below 1,500 microliters. BEN is a diagnosis that was created when African American populations were found to have lower neutrophil counts compared to white Americans in the 1940s. However, this lower white blood cell count was simply relative and did not confer an increased risk of infection. Today, many Black American patients who would benefit from receiving clozapine are either not offered it, consequent to physician fear of BEN, or forgo it themselves when told they will need invasive blood draws and frequent monitoring.

The preconceived correlation between Black Americans and BEN has also affected breast cancer treatment in African American patients. Studies demonstrate there are breast cancer survival disparities between Black Americans and white Americans. Aside from socioeconomic status and health care differences, the discrepancies may be related to the fact that, out of concern for lower baseline absolute neutrophil count, physicians more frequently reduce doses and discontinue chemotherapy treatments in African Americans, in turn, lowering survival rates.

It is important to note that, when compared to other cancer patients, BEN patients are not at an increased risk of infection or neutropenic fever after initiation of chemotherapy. So, these race-based clinical decisions may be doing more harm than good. Altogether, using race as a medical tool in a patient's HPI has social, historical, and medical consequences and needs to be rethought.

Many physicians believe it is crucial to incorporate race into a patient's note. They argue that it is an important medical indicator, a convenient stand-in for genetics. But, if physicians are truly trying to discern if patients are carriers of genetic allelic variants that cause severe medication reactions (e.g., antiepileptic drugs causing toxic epidermal necrolysis in people with HLA-B*15:02 alleles) or put them at an immensely higher disease risk (e.g., the Duffy antigen/receptor chemokine gene and neutropenia), then genetic mapping should be used in high-risk patients. Although genotyping is a more costly option, using racial suspicions to deny patients gold standard treatments–that have better health outcomes and side effect profiles–is hardly cost-effective. Most importantly, this type of gradated treatment is inhumane.

Some medical professionals already recognize the lack of basis for employing race-based medicine. For instance, the *New England Journal of Medicine*'s highly regarded weekly section "Case Records of the Massachusetts General Hospital" does not include race in the first sentence of patients' histories or really at all. In Canada, a country with immense racial diversity and good health outcomes, neither the *Canadian Medical Association Journal* nor the *Canadian Journal of Surgery* reports race in their case reports. To be clear, a "color-blind" approach is not ideal either. The understanding of race is important for health disparities research. Yet, when it is collected in research settings, it can be done in a self-identified, consistent and consensual manner.

Ultimately, medicine is reaching a tipping point. The National Kidney Foundation recently announced that it would no longer be using race as part of its eGFR calculation for kidney function and transplant urgency. Changes like these illustrate that these are not just radical arguments embedded in social justice. They are sound, scientific arguments embedded in evidence-based medicine, with the goal of providing the best patient care possible at their core.

Together, the genetic inaccuracy, lack of patient self-identification and biased use of racial labels by providers when writing HPIs make it more likely to perpetuate racism than optimize patient health. In general, noting a patient's race in the first line of their history is not clinically useful in understanding their disease or creating a treatment plan. Factors like a patient's family history, insurance status, work, transportation, nutrition and housing situation are more medically indicative. If the medical profession is serious about addressing racial health disparities, it may need to rethink some of its fundamental tools. Civil rights activist Audre Lorde wrote, "The master's tools will never dismantle the master's house." If we continue to unquestioningly use tools developed by the mostly white forefathers of the medical profession, we may never actually change racial health disparities.

About the Author

Ashley Andreou is a medical student at Georgetown University.

Antifatness in the Surgical Setting

By Ashley Andreou

It was 6:30 A.M., and I was getting ready to head down to the operating room (OR) for the first case of the day: an abdominal wall hernia repair. In preparation for the case, I logged on to the electronic health record portal and read through the patient's medical history and the preoperative notes written by the surgical team. In many of the physician notes, the first line noted the patient's body mass index (BMI) of 41. The patient's ventral hernia was estimated to be 30 centimeters by 20 cm, one of the largest hernias ever repaired by the surgeon I was working with. The CT scan showed sections of the large intestine protruding through the hernia, which posed a high risk for bowel twisting, which can lead to perforation and sepsis or tissue deoxygenation and necrosis. The patient's condition had reached a critical point.

I ventured down to the OR and located the CT and MRI images, as part of my medical student role of assisting the nursing and scrub technicians in prepping the OR prior to surgery. I projected the scans onto the large screen TVs hanging in the OR to help the surgeons better visualize the anatomy and their approach. As I pulled up the images, the team in the room erupted in shock. How could someone let a hernia get this bad before seeking medical consultation, they wondered. And others couldn't believe that someone could live with such a large defect and not want it fixed for cosmetic purposes. After rolling the patient into the OR and moving her onto the operating table, the team began to prep the surgical site. As she drifted off into a state of sedation, medical staff in the room could not stop talking about her BMI. The comments were unrelenting throughout the five-hour procedure, as people took turns gawking at the gaping hole in the patient's abdomen. Two of the largest pieces of Strattice biologic mesh made by the supplier were sewn together to repair the hernia. The estimated cost of the mesh alone was $30,000.

As the surgery ended, I couldn't stop thinking about the obvious, yet ironic, connection between the weight comments from the health care team and why the patient procrastinated before getting the surgery. Why would *anyone* want to interact with a medical system that looked at them in such a derogatory way?

Antifatness is socially ingrained and virtually inescapable. Pop culture idolizes thinness. The Centers for Disease Control and Prevention created an alarmist "obesity epidemic" based on exaggerated data that haven't held up. Like everyone else in society who is socially conditioned to this bias, clinicians are not exempt from harboring antifatness. In a recent study, 24 percent of physicians stated they were uncomfortable having friends in larger bodies, and 18 percent admitted they felt disgusted when treating a patient with a high BMI. This is upsetting, yet unsurprising considering that few programs actively train health care providers against this cognitive bias.

Abundant research demonstrates that "obesity" is not really a choice and is often a product of systemic inequity. The crux of this research explores the multiple systems that underpin weight: food insecurity, housing insecurity, poverty-induced scarcity mindset, medications, diseases, lack of education, mental health issues and chronic stress among them.

Many researchers and scholars have exposed the pervasiveness of antifatness culture, but some of the most prominent actors in maintaining this culture have not been discussed. Surgeons are central to dismantling the problems of antifat bias in health care, and that requires addressing aspects of surgeons' training and day-to-day tasks that may make them more prone to this cognitive bias.

Weight bias is heightened and reinforced in the surgical setting, where surgeries on higher BMI individuals take more time, cost more money and have an increased risk of complications. Antifatness attitudes and behaviors may be higher among surgeons partly as a result of the lack of filter people may have when the patient is sedated. The increased time and care required in these cases can be difficult for surgeons, whose time and care are already strained given staff shortages. Together, these factors may lead surgeons to express their frustration through comments about the patient's body.

In addition, professional culture and training are different for surgeons. Primary care physicians' training may focus more on upstream factors contributing to care, including being taught about social determinants of health and multifactorial causes of the patients' conditions. In contrast, surgeons–who on average spend 3,963 hours of training honing a complex motor and visuospatial skill–may naturally focus more on the procedural task at hand rather than the factors contributing to their patient's condition. Ultimately, the everyday demands of a surgeon's job may make them less likely to think critically about antifatness when providing their day-to-day care. Yet, to provide optimal patient care, it is equally important for surgeons to work against weight stigma.

Surgeons are often the physicians who spend the most time in the hospital. As such, they play a vital role in forming the culture in the OR and hospital at large, and their understanding of weight bias and its associated behaviors is critical to counteracting pervasive weight stigma among health care providers. Post-surgery, many higher-weight patients will require intensive care, continual follow-up and long-term treatment adherence. Patients with a higher weight are also 12 times more likely to have a complication requiring extended hospitalization and continued interface with their surgical team. Surgeons must confront their own weight bias to build positive ongoing partnerships with patients.

A culture of antifatness among surgeons leads to compounding negative impacts on individual patients and the health system. Studies show weight bias from providers is palpable for patients. Patients can sense the lack of dignity and respect in providers' attitudes and, in turn, may choose not to interact with the system that degrades them. Many clinicians turn weight loss into an ultimatum for patients rather than focusing on building their trust, understanding contributing factors and partnering with them to make incremental lifestyle modifications possible. Altogether this can harm patients' self-worth and rapport with providers.

When providers alienate patients who first touch the health care system, through poor care or rapport, these patients are more likely to not resurface until reaching a critical health point, as with the hernia repair case discussed above. Research suggests that providers spend less time with larger patients, provide a lower quality of care and misdiagnose larger patients more frequently.

Antifatness is often a more socially acceptable masquerade for anti-Blackness. The Department of Health and Human Services reports that about four out of five African American women are overweight or obese, and Black Americans were 1.3 times more likely to be obese compared to white Americans. This intersection allows covert ways to harm Black and brown bodies.

Ultimately, the biases and behaviors that maintain antifatness need to change. Potential avenues for change include creating systemwide education, amending medical documentation, reframing patient conversations and advocating for upstream policies that increase access. A health provider's goal should be health–vital statistics, lab results, symptom reduction, time spent exercising, mental health–not thinness. There are health consequences to obesity, but the current BMI-focused approach is not the best way to capture a person's current health status. Lack of education among medical professionals is perpetuating antifatness. A health systemwide training should be developed to educate health care providers and shift conscious and unconscious attitudes.

Providers should also make a habit of noting diet and exercise in social history, as opposed to collapsing these factors into BMI. They could partner with patients and connect them with community resources to enable them to meet their health goals of lower blood pressure or better cardiovascular health. Providers can also focus on evidence-based methods, such as educating patients about nutrition, increasing access to food or exercise, discussing weight-loss surgery or medication and employing motivational interviewing. Understanding the multifactorial nature of weight and taking a patient-centered approach early on can ensure patients feel supported and empowered to achieve optimal health outcomes. This affirmative type of partnership will encourage patients to return to the health care system and invest in the provider-patient relationship and health goals. Providers must internalize the complexity of weight, learn how to utilize alternative health markers and even advocate for policies that reduce food deserts. Surgeons may read the above action items and write them off as tasks reserved for primary care physicians. But practicing unbiased medicine is possible. In one promising model, hospitals in Canada have recently launched a surgical prehabilitation program and toolkit that helps surgeons and their patients work on hypertension, hyperglycemia, hyperlipidemia and cardiovascular health.

Recent movements around self-love and body acceptance are important, but they cannot replace the work that needs to be done by the people who manifest antifatness bias. America does not have an obesity epidemic; it has an unhealthiness epidemic. Yet the worse health outcomes compared to countries with similar economies are just as much a product of antifatness as they are of fatness. Through shame and blame, antifatness may be contributing to obesity and exacerbating poor health. Until surgeons and other health care providers choose to be a part of the solution to antifatness, then they will be part of the problem.

This is an opinion and analysis article, and the views expressed by the author or authors are not necessarily those of Scientific American.

About the Author

Ashley Andreou is a medical student at Georgetown University.

GLOSSARY

algorithm A set of specific ordered instructions, often for a computer.

angina A condition of chronic chest pain.

autoimmune A condition where the body produces antibodies against its own cells or tissues.

biologic therapy A medical treatment that uses components of living organisms to combat disease.

body mass index A commonly used measure of obesity calculated using one's height and weight, currently controversial in assessing the health of larger people.

disparity A difference in outcome or treatment between two or more groups.

dopamine A neurochemical associated with feelings of pleasure and well-being.

endocrine Relating to the hormones in the body and the glands that secrete them.

exosuit A powered and/or armored suit worn to enhance specific physical capacities.

in utero The period when an organism is developing in the uterus.

invertebrate A group of animal species characterized by a lack of backbone.

multiplier effect When the impact of an action is greater than the action itself.

origami A traditional Japanese art of folding paper, often studied for its applications in mathematics and engineering.

plasticity Ability to adapt or be molded, often described as a feature of the brain.

polymer A synthetic or natural substance made of large molecules comprised of smaller replicating components.

predation When an organism kills and eats another for sustenance.

proliferation The rapid and widespread increase of something.

regimen A recommended course of medicine, diet, or exercise prescribed as a component of medical or wellness treatment.

reimburse To repay money that has been spent or lost.

reproducibility crisis A dilemma faced in some research disciplines, where findings in a study cannot be reproduced by other researchers.

shaman A social role played in some societies, where a person may have special access to spiritual insights, as well as techniques in healing, fortune-telling, and story-telling.

socioeconomic status Social or class position as determined by wealth, power, culture, education, or other factors.

FURTHER INFORMATION

"Medical Devices." World Health Organization, https://www.who.int/health-topics/medical-devices.

"What Is Public Health?," American Public Health Assocation, https://www.apha.org/what-is-public-health.

Fitzharris, Lindsey. "How Ether Transformed Surgery from a Race against the Clock." *Scientific American,* October 1, 2017, https://www.scientificamerican.com/article/how-ether-transformed-surgery-from-a-race-against-the-clock/.

Kaushal, Amit, Russ Altman, and Curt Langlotz. "Health Care AI Systems Are Biased." *Scientific American*, November 17, 2020, https://www.scientificamerican.com/article/health-care-ai-systems-are-biased/.

Maron, Dina Fine. "How a Transgender Woman Could Get Pregnant." *Scientific American*, June 15, 2016, https://www.scientificamerican.com/article/how-a-transgender-woman-could-get-pregnant/.

McDonough, Megan. "A Black Mother's Loss Explains Why U.S. Maternal Health Care Is Broken." *Scientific American*, October 20, 2022, https://www.scientificamerican.com/video/a-black-mothers-loss-explains-why-u-s-maternal-healthcare-is-broken/.

Wong, Kate. "Mother Nature's Medicine Cabinet." *Scientific American*, April 9, 2001, https://www.scientificamerican.com/article/mother-natures-medicine-c/.

CITATIONS

1.1 An Innovative Robotic Exosuit Boosts both Walking and Running by Jeremy Hsu (August 16, 2019); 1.2 A New Type of Visual Prosthesis by Stephen L. Macknik (August 27, 2019); 1.3 The Surgical Singularity Is Approaching by Sandip S. Panesar (December 27, 2018); 1.4 Neck-Zapping Gadget Reduced All-Nighter Fatigue in New Study by Maddie Bender (June 10, 2021); 1.5 Experimental Brain Implant Could Personalize Depression Therapy by Gary Stix (October 4, 2021); 1.6 AI in Medicine Is Overhyped by Visar Berisha, Julie Liss (October 19, 2022); 2.1 Can Hearing Be Restored by Making the Brain More Childlike? by Mo Costandi (June 29, 2017); 2.2 How Virtual Reality Will Transform Medicine by Claudia Wallis (February 1, 2019); 2.3 Can 3-D Printing Produce Lung and Liver Tissue for Transplants? by Starre Vartan (May 6, 2019); 2.4 The Case for Fewer Heart Procedures by Claudia Wallis (February 1, 2020); 2.5 A Breakthrough in Genetic Medicine for Rare Diseases by Lydia Denworth (March 1, 2020); 3.1 A Better Pill—Internal Delivery Devices May Help Patients Take Their Medicine by Knvul Sheikh (February 8, 2019); 3.2 How Nanotech Powers Precision Medicine by Robert Langer (June 12, 2019); 3.3 Tiny, Tumbling Origami Robots Could Help with Targeted Drug Delivery by Fionna M. D. Samuels (June 14, 2022); 3.4 Hope for New Drugs Arises from the Sea by Stephanie Stone (August 1, 2022); 4.1 Drug Developers Take a Second Look at Herbal Medicines by Brendan Borrell (June 1, 2014); 4.2 Traditional Medicine from Southern Mexico Offers Help with Addiction by Peter H. Addy, Ana Elda Maqueda (August 11, 2015); 4.3 Anti-Vaxxers Are Here to Stay by Beth S. Linas (February 28, 2019); 4.4 The World Health Organization Gives the Nod to Traditional Chinese Medicine. Bad Idea by The Editors of *Scientific American* (April 1, 2019); 5.1 Maternal Health Care Is Disappearing in Rural America by Dina Fine Maron (February 15, 2017); 5.2 Abortion Bans Based on So-Called "Science" Are Fraudulent by Nicole M. Baran, Gretchen Goldman, Jane Zelikova on (August 21, 2019); 5.3 What the Science on Gender-Affirming Care for Transgender Kids Really Shows by Heather Boerner (May 12, 2022); 5.4 What Scientists Are Learning about Women's Health from Other Female Animals by Barbara Natterson-Horowitz (March 1, 2023); 6.1 Potential Inequities in New Medical Technologies by Eric B. Kmiec, Jonathan Marron (March 28, 2020); 6.2 Inequality before Birth Contributes to Health Inequality in Adults by Janet Currie (October 1, 2020); 6.3 A Tool Doctors Use Every Day Can Perpetuate Medical Racism by Ashley Andreou (June 7, 2021); 6.4 Antifatness in the Surgical Setting by Ashley Andreou (May 26, 2022).

Each author biography was accurate at the time the article was originally published.

INDEX

A

abortion bans, dangers of, 104–110
alternative medicine, 75–84, 85–89, 94–96
antisense oligonucleotides (ASOs) treatment for rare diseases, 44–54
anti-vaxxers, increase in, 90–93
artificial intelligence (AI) in medicine, 8–11, 12–14, 19–22, 23–25
  problems with accuracy, 26–29

C

COVID-19, 20, 66–67, 70–71, 132, 133, 141, 143, 145

D

depression, brain implant for treating, 23–25
drug development and delivery
  drugs sourced from the sea, 66–73
  internal delivery devices, 56–59
  precision medicine using nanotechnology, 60–62
  tiny origami robots for drug delivery, 63–65

E

electricity, low-voltage to keep people awake, 19–22
exposure therapy, 35

G

gender dysphoria, 111, 114

H

hearing, restoring by inhibiting adenosine signaling, 31–33
heart procedures, the case for fewer, 41–43
herbal medicines, 75–84, 85–89, 94, 95

I

inequality in medicine
  antifatness in surgical settings, 150–154
  before birth and into adulthood, 132–144
  medical racism, 132, 145–149
  potential for in new technologies, 128–131

L

language learning, improving, 31–33

M

marine environments, sourcing drugs from, 66–73
maternal health care, 107–108, 132, 136, 139– 141, 143
  in rural America, 98–103
metabolic cost, 8–9

N

nanotechnology and medicine, 60–¬62
National Institutes of Health, 12, 121, 130

O

organ transplants and 3-D printing, 37–40

P

post-traumatic stress disorder (PTSD), 34–35, 36

R

racism, medical, 132, 145–149
reproductive and sexual health, 98–103, 104–110, 111–117, 118–126
reverse pharmacology, 76, 78, 81–82
RNA
  RNA interference (RNAi), 47–49
  therapy, 61
robotic exosuit to aid walking and running, 8–11
robotic surgery, 15–18

S

SOMA pill, 56–59
spinal muscular atrophy (SMA), 44–46, 50–51, 53–54
substance abuse, traditional medicine to help with, 85–89
surgical singularity, 17–18

T

telemedicine, 61, 102
3-D printing of lung and liver tissue for transplants, 37–40
Traditional Chinese Medicine, 94–96
transgender kids, gender-affirming care for, 111–117

V

vagus nerve stimulation, 19–22
virtual reality (VR), transforming medicine, 34–36
visual prosthetics, 12–14

W

women's health, learning about from female animals, 118–126
World Health Organization (WHO), 91, 94–96